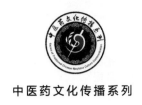

中医药文化传播系列

读故事 识本草
——中药入门读本

A BILINGUAL INTRODUCTION TO
CHINESE HERBAL MEDICINE

毛国强　谭秀敏　李兰兰◎主编

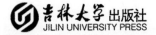
吉林大学出版社
JILIN UNIVERSITY PRESS

图书在版编目（CIP）数据

读故事　识本草：中药入门读本 / 毛国强，
谭秀敏，李兰兰主编. —长春：吉林大学出版
社，2019.6
　　ISBN 978-7-5692-4959-0

　　Ⅰ. ①读… Ⅱ. ①毛… ②谭… ③李… Ⅲ. ①中草药
－基本知识－汉、英 Ⅳ. ①R282

中国版本图书馆CIP数据核字（2019）第119082号

书　　名	读故事　识本草——中药入门读本	
	DU GUSHI　SHI BENCAO——ZHONGYAO RUMEN DUBEN	
作　　者	毛国强　谭秀敏　李兰兰　主编	
策划编辑	刘明明	
责任编辑	曲　楠	
责任校对	赵雪君	
装帧设计	中尚图	
出版发行	吉林大学出版社	
社　　址	长春市人民大街4059号	
邮政编码	130021	
发行电话	0431-89580028/29/21	
网　　址	http://www.jlup.com.cn	
电子邮箱	jdcbs@jlu.edu.cn	
印　　刷	河北盛世彩捷印刷有限公司	
开　　本	880mm×1230mm　1/32	
印　　张	9.25	
字　　数	150千字	
版　　次	2019年6月　第1版	
印　　次	2019年6月　第1次	
书　　号	ISBN 978-7-5692-4959-0	
定　　价	59.80元	

本书编写组成员

主　编：毛国强　谭秀敏　李兰兰

副主编：张　坚　赵习群　马　琳

编　委：刘　佳　李先宽　李　鹏

　　　　李　静　张　庆　陈志娟

总　序

　　中医药学源远流长，它凝聚了中华民族宇宙观、生命观、人生观的精华，同时也吸收了其他学科的知识成果。几千年来，硕果累累，名医辈出，一直守护着中华儿女的身心健康。中医药的价值不仅体现在精深的医学知识，还体现在丰厚的文化内涵。中医药文化具有强大的生命力和持续的创造力，是理解和传承中华优秀传统文化的重要抓手。

　　《中华人民共和国中医药法》的颁布、国务院发表《中国的中医药》白皮书，标志着中医药发展上升为国家战略，中医药事业进入新的历史发展时期。习近平总书记多次对中医药给予高度评价，他在给中国中医科学院60周年院庆的贺信中指出"中医药学凝聚着深邃的哲学智慧和中华民族几千年的健康养生理念及其实践经验，是中国古代科学的瑰宝，也是打开中华文明宝库的钥匙。深入研究和科学总结中医药学对丰富世界医学事业、推进生命科学研究具有积极意义"，同时希望广大中医药工作者"切实把中医药这一祖先留给我们的宝贵财富继承好、发展好、利用好，在建设健康中国、实现中国梦的伟大征程中谱写新的篇章"。2017年1月，中共中央办公厅、国务院办公厅印发了《关于实施中华优秀传统文化传承发展工程的意见》。中医药文化是中华优秀传统文化的重要组成部分，我们要通过多种形式向广大青少年传授基本的中医药文化知识，使他们了解中医药在日常生活、传统习俗、文学艺术等方方面面的文化蕴含，在他们心中播撒下热爱中医药文化的种子。

　　可喜的是，在天津市卫生健康委、天津市中医药管理局的高度重视下和大力支持下，2017和2018两年多时间里，天津中医药大学获得多个中医药文化研究方面的立项。其中，"中医药文化进校园"项目组负责人毛国强教授带领项目组成员，在开展中医药文化传播研究的同时，还开拓思路深入全市近20多所中小学试点校，开展了多项中医文化推广活动，包括中医药文化知识宣讲、中医保健讲座、中药囊制作，并组织大中小学生参观百年老字号中药厂，参加中医药文化主题夏令营、中医药主题诗词音乐朗诵会等，将中医药的知识传授与文化传承与传播活动很好地融合在一起。项目开展的两年时间里，全市数千名中小学生参与其中，许多学生表现出对中医药文化浓厚的兴趣，各种活动也在社会上引起较好的反响。为了满足青少年进一步了解中医药知识的需求，项目组组织邀请相关专家多次研讨，以天津中医药大学相关专业教师为主，在广泛吸纳了中小学教育专家、师生意见建议基础上，编写了《中医药文化精选读本》（小学版和中学版）。其中小学版读本立足小学生阅读特点，通过一个个小故事，辅以卡通漫画形象，讲述故事里蕴含的中医药文化知识以及浅显易懂的中医文化哲理，图文并茂，形象传神。在不增加孩子们负担的情况下，激发他们对中医药知识的好奇心和求知欲。中学版读本遵循中学生的认知规律，以通俗的科普小故事为载体，通过"识人体，解中医""读课本，学中药""观生活，明中医""体民俗，感中医""读名篇，叙中医"等五个章节传递中医药文化知识，化繁为简，深入浅出，培养中学生对于中医药文化的感知与热爱。作为此书的总主编，我曾多次参加这套读本的编写会议，编写组先后6次邀请全国及天津市各方面专家召开研讨论证、评审会，对读本构架、内容设计广泛征询意见，历时两年对文字内容、配图形式、板式设计等进行10多次修改、完善，精心组织、精细打磨、精益求精，力求既科学严谨通俗、又可读好看。相信，这套面向青少年的中医药文化读本会对他们了解中医药文化起到帮助作用，也会培养更多对中医药文化感兴趣的未来"中医药人"。

除了这两册面向青少年的读本以外，首批"中医药文化传播系列"中，面向中老年读者的《中医名家谈节气养生与文化》是在《中老年时报》颐寿专栏刊稿的基础上扩展而成，倾注了许多中医大家名家的心血。

书中有对三位中国工程院院士、九位国医大师、十多位名中医的访谈，他们用通俗易懂的话语、生动形象的表述，为读者悉心讲授节气养生的要诀。如此多的大家、名家为老百姓普及中医养生、健康常识，在全国中医科普类书籍中是开先河的。除养生宝典外，编著者十分用心，还汇集了与节气有关的民俗、谚语、古诗词等深厚的节气文化内涵，相信读者定会开卷有益，受益匪浅。

中医药文化不仅是我国的优秀传统文化，还是全人类的精神财富。新形势下，我们应该讲好中医的"中国故事"，做好中医药文化国际传播这篇大文章。本套书中有两本以外国留学生和来华工作、旅行者为主要受众对象的书也同样值得关注。《中医药文化概览》为全英文读本，以中医零基础的外国人士为目标读者，面向来华工作、学习、生活、旅游并对中医药文化感兴趣的外国朋友。《读故事，识本草——中药入门读本》则是双语读本，目标读者是对中药感兴趣的外国人，及来华读书的留学生。该书介绍了五十种常见常用的中药，以及这些中药背后的有趣故事，还介绍了药材在食品、养生、化妆品、园林绿化等方面的利用价值。

作为在全国有影响力的中医药类高校，天津中医药大学在传承和发展中医药文化上责无旁贷。特别是在贯彻全国教育大会精神、建设国家"双一流"高校的契机下，文化传承与创新板块成为建设的一个重要内容。而文化的传承与活力需要动态的传播来体现，平台和载体的建设尤为重要。2017年，我校成立了中医药文化研究与传播中心，成立仅一年就成果颇丰，2018年即升级为天津市级机构，由天津市卫健委与我校共建。该中心落户在文化与健康传播学院，它们发挥人文学院优势，联合中医学院、中药学院及社会力量，不仅开展了10多项中医文化研究，还组织了形式多样的中医药文化主题大众传播活动。这一套书即是其中的成果之一。

我由衷希望这套书在传承和弘扬中医药文化方面发挥积极作用，成为国人乃至全世界了解和学习中医药文化的好帮手。

这套书的编写和出版，得到了众多中医药人、社会各界的帮助和支持。参与编写工作的专家、老师、同学们十分投入和认真，圆满地完成了预定任务。

尤其令我感动的是，德高望重，才艺双馨，在海内外享有盛誉，已经94岁高龄的古典诗词大家叶嘉莹先生，欣然为《中医名家谈节气养生与文化》一书撰写推介感言。在此，一并表示深深的敬意和衷心感谢。

中医药文化要从中国走向世界，要以传统面向未来。任重而道远，让我们一起努力！

中国工程院院士

天津中医药大学校长

2019年5月于天津团泊湖畔

张伯礼　中国工程院院士，全国名中医，中医内科学专家，天津中医药大学校长，国务院政府特殊津贴专家，国家有突出贡献中青年专家；国家"重大新药创制"重大专项技术副总师，国务院医政咨询专家委员会委员，教育部医学教育专家委员会副主任；参加国家中医药现代化顶层设计；参加起草了《中医现代化科技发展战略》《中药现代化发展纲要》等文件；作为全国人大代表提出《发展中医药健康服务业规划》等数十项议案和建议；提出并推动了《中医药法》颁布实施。

前　言

　　我国的中医药文化源远流长，凝聚了几千年来劳动人民的经验与智慧，是中华民族的重要瑰宝，是向全世界展示中华优秀文化的一扇窗口，也是沟通中西方文化的一座桥梁。我国"一带一路"倡议的提出和实施，为中医药国际化带来了重大机遇。同时，青少年是传承与传播优秀中华传统文化的生力军，肩负着在未来继承和弘扬中医药文化的重任。在此背景下，向大众尤其是青少年普及中医药文化势在必行。

　　为了普及中医药知识，弘扬中医药文化，增强文化自信，并且深入贯彻中共中央办公厅、国务院办公厅《关于实施中华优秀传统文化传承发展工程的意见》以及国务院《中医药发展战略规划纲要（2016-2030年）》精神，我们特此编写了《读故事，识本草——中药入门读本》一书。本书为双语读本，目标读者为广大热爱传统文化的青少年，以及来华工作、学习、生活和旅游，对中医药文化感兴趣的外国人。本书首先介绍了中药的一些常识，然后着重介绍了五十种生活中常见和常用的中药，包括这些中药的相关知识和趣味故事。为了突出中药资源的综合利用，还涉及了一些药材在其他方面的利用价值，如在食品、养生、化妆品和园林绿化等方面做了简单阐述，希望能抛砖引玉，提高大家对中药文化的兴趣。

　　本书按照中药的生物属性和药用部位进行编排，目的是希望大家对中药本身有一个真实客观的认识，然后在此基础上再了解其功效主治。同时，本书力求图文并茂，增强读本的直观性和可读性，使广大读者对我国的中药文化有一个初步的了解，能认识一些常见常用的中草药，在生活中能利用所学的中药知识解决一些简单问题。

此书作为天津市中医药文化研究与传播中心、天津中医药大学文化与健康传播学院策划编写的"中医药文化系列丛书"其中之一，得到了中国工程院院士、天津中医药大学校长张伯礼教授的大力支持。天津市卫生健康委、市中医药管理局相关领导也对此书给予了支持和帮助，一并表示感谢。

在本书的编写过程中，因为水平有限，难免会出现一些疏漏和不足之处，恳请各位专家、学者、同行和读者朋友们给予批评指正，并提出宝贵的意见和建议。

编者

Preface

With a long history, the Traditional Chinese Medicine (TCM) is the result of the experience and wisdom of Chinese people in the past thousands of years. It is a treasure of the Chinese nation, a window through which the excellent Chinese culture is shown to the world, and also a bridge between Chinese and Western cultures. At present, the proposal and implementation of the Belt and Road Initiative brings great opportunities for the internationalization of TCM. Meanwhile, the teenagers are the new force to inherit and promote the excellent traditional Chinese culture, and they will also shoulder the important task of inheriting and promoting the culture of TCM in the future. Under this background, it is imperative to spread culture of TCM to the public, especially the teenagers.

Therefore, in order to spread the knowledge and culture of TCM, enhance our cultural self-confidence, and thoroughly implement the spirit of "Suggestions on Implementation of Projects to Promote and Develop Excellent Traditional Chinese Culture" issued by the General Office of the CPC Central Committee and the General Office of the State Council, as well as the spirit of "National Outline of the Strategic Plan for the Development of Traditional Chinese Medicine (2016– 2030)" issued by the State Council, we hereby compile this book entitled *A Bilingual Introduction to Chinese Herbal Medicine*. The targeting readers of this bilingual book include the adolescents, who are fond of traditional culture, as well as foreigners, who work, study, live and travel in China or who are interested in the culture of Chinese herbal medicine. The book firstly introduces some basic knowledge of Chinese herbal medicine, and then introduces 50 kinds of Chinese herbal medicines commonly seen and commonly used in daily life, including the related knowledge and interesting stories of these herbs. In order to highlight the comprehensive utilization of Chinese medicine resources, this book also includes the application of these medicines in some other areas, such as food, health care, cosmetics, gardening and so on, hoping to inspire the reader's interest in Chinese herbal medicine culture.

This book is arranged according to the biological attributes and medicinal parts of these medicines. We hope that readers will have an objective understanding of these Chinese herbal medicines, and then on this basis, readers can further understand their efficacy and indications. At the same time, the book also includes many pictures to make it more visual and readable. After reading the book, the readers can have a preliminary understanding of the culture of Chinese herbal medicine, and thus can learn some Chinese herbal medicines. Besides, the readers can also use the medical knowledge that they have learned to solve some simple problems in life.

As one of the series of books about TCM culture planned and organized by TCM Culture Research and Communication Center of Tianjin and College of Culture and Health Communication of Tianjin University of Traditional Chinese Medicine, this book has received strong support from Professor Zhang Boli, academician of the Chinese Academy of Engineering and president of Tianjin University of Traditional Chinese Medicine. Relevant leaders of Tianjin Municipal Health Commission and Tianjin Administration of Traditional Chinese Medicine also gave much support and help to this book. We are deeply grateful to all of them.

However, the book might be imperfect due to the limited ability of the writers. We would like to invite experts, peers, teachers, students and readers to give your valuable comments and suggestions.

Writers

目录
Contents

第一章　中药常识
Basic knowledge of Chinese herbal medicine

1

第二章　五十种常见中药介绍
An introduction to fifty common Chinese herbal medicines

第三章　中药文化
Culture of Chinese Herbal Medicine

第一章　中药常识

Basic knowledge of Chinese herbal medicine

一、什么是中药？ / What is Chinese herbal medicine?

　　中国的药文化有着数千年的悠久历史和丰厚的底蕴。我们的祖国幅员辽阔，地大物博，拥有种类繁多的天然中药资源，几千年来，我国人民对这些宝贵资源进行开发和利用，这些宝贵的中药资源也一直是我国劳动人民防病治病的主要武器，保障了人民的健康和中华民族的繁衍昌盛，同时也推动了我国医药学的发展。

　　那么到底什么是中药呢？我们现在所说的中药是相对于西药而言的，其实在古代，我们的祖先并没有"中药"这一概念。由于中药基本以植物药为主，所以古代人们就把"中药"叫作"本草"。19世纪时西药传入我国，为了把我国传统药与西药区别开来，就将传统药称为"中药"。简而言之，中药就是指在中医理论指导下使用的药物，用于预防、治疗、诊断疾病，并具有康复和保健的作用。中药主要来源于天然药及其加工品，包括植物药、动物药、矿物药及部分化学、生物制品类药物。

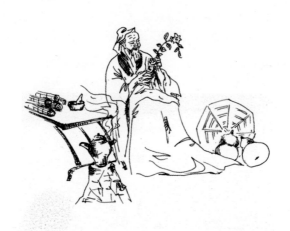

Chinese medicine culture has a long history and rich heritage. China is a large country with a wide range of natural medical resources. For thousands of years, the Chinese people have exploited and utilized these precious resources as the weapon to prevent and treat various diseases, which guaranteed the health of the people and the prosperity of the Chinese nation, and also promoted the development of medical science in ancient China.

What exactly is Chinese herbal medicine? This name is the result of the introduction of Western medicine into China. Actually, there was no concept of "Chinese medicine" in ancient China. Since the vast majority of Chinese herbal medicines are botanical medicines, people in ancient China called them "Ben Cao" (which means herbal medicine). In the 19th century, the Western medicine was introduced into China. In order to distinguish the Chinese medicine from the Western medicine, the traditional medicine of China was then called "Chinese medicine". In short, Chinese herbal medicine refers to the medicines used with the guidance of TCM theory for the prevention, treatment and diagnosis of diseases, and they have the functions of rehabilitation and health care. Chinese herbal medicines, which mainly come from natural resources and their processed products, include botanical medicine, animal medicine, mineral medicine and some chemical and biological products.

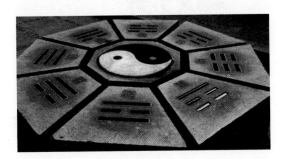

二、中药的分类 / Categorization of Chinese herbal medicine

　　中药是一个十分庞大的家族，根据近年的统计，总数约在一万余种，常用的中药也多达四五百种。因此，如果按一定的标准把这些中药分门别类，那么我们学习、研究和应用起来就容易多了。根据目的与侧重点的不同，中药分类的方法有很多，最常用的分类方法主要有以下两种。

　　按药物功能分类——解表药、泻下药、清热药、理气药和滋补药、活血化瘀药等。

　　按药用部位分类——植物类、动物类和矿物类，植物类中药再依药用部位分为根、根茎、茎木、皮、叶、花、果实、种子和全草等。

　　这些分类方法各有优缺点，究竟采用哪一种分类方法，主要取决于我们的目的和要求。比如，按药物功能分类，有利于学习和研究中药的作用和用途，按药用部位分类有助于快速认识中药的自然属性和性状特征，有利于药材的鉴定。

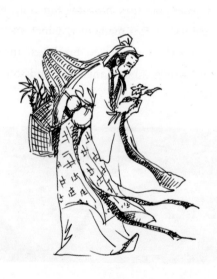

The Chinese herbal medicine is a huge family which contains over 10,000 kinds of medicines according to the statistics in recent years. Even the number of the most commonly used medicines is up to over four hundred. Therefore, if we classify these Chinese medicines based on certain standards, it will be much easier for us to study, research and apply them. According to different purposes, there are many categorization methods, while the following two are the most popular ones.

The categorization based on functions-such as relieving exterior syndrome, purgation, clearing heat, regulating qi, nourishing, activating blood circulation to dissipate blood stasis, etc.

The categorization based on medicinal parts-such as botanical medicine, animal medicine and mineral medicine. Botanical medicine is further classified according to different parts including root, rhizome, stem, wood, bark, leaf, flower, fruit, seed, and whole herb, etc.

Different categorization methods have their own advantages and disadvantages. What method we adopt mainly depends on our purpose and requirements. For example, the classification based on functions is convenient for people to study the functions and usage of the medicines, while the classification based on medicinal parts can help people to understand the natural attributes and characteristics of the medicines, and is conducive to the identification of the Chinese herbal medicines.

三、中药的"四气五味" / Four natures and five flavors of Chinese herbal medicine

中国古代的历代医家在医疗实践中逐步探索出中药的性能。而中药治病，就是利用每种药物的不同性能，来恢复和调整我们身体各脏腑的功能，纠正人体内的阴阳失衡。

"气"是指药物的性质。就像一年四季的气候各不相同，中药有四气，又称四性，即寒、热、温、凉。这里所说的"寒热温凉"可不是我们平时所说的温度，而是指药物的性质，是根据人体对药物的反应以及药物的治疗效果而总结出来的。比如，有些疾病属于热证，就需要用寒凉性的中药来治疗，如菊花、黄连、百合和薄荷等，这些药具有清热、解毒和泻火等功效；有些疾病属于寒证，就需要温热性的中药来治疗，如人参、当归和防风等，这类药物具有温中、散寒等作用。

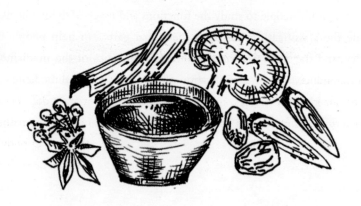

"味"是指药物的味道。五味就是药物的五种基本的味道——辛、甘、酸、苦、咸。

辛：辛味药具有发散、行气和活血的作用，适用于外感表证、气滞血瘀及风寒痹症等。如半夏、紫苏、白芷和川芎等。

甘：甘味药具有调和脾胃、补益气血及缓急止痛的作用，适用于机体虚弱等症，并能调和药性，常如人参、党参、甘草和枸杞子等。

酸：酸味药具有收敛、固涩的作用，适用于体虚多汗、久泻肠滑、遗精滑精及尿频失禁等，如五味子、山楂、金樱子和覆盆子等。

苦：苦味药具有清热解毒、燥湿、泻火和通便的作用，适用于热证、湿热及痈肿疮疡等，如黄连、大黄和苦杏仁等。

咸：咸味药具有软坚散结、泻下通便等作用，如蜈蚣、牡蛎和芒硝等。

Ancient Chinese doctors have gradually discovered the properties of Chinese herbal medicines in their medical practice. Actually, the reason why Chinese herbal medicine can cure diseases is because the different properties of these medicines can help restore and adjust the functions of our internal organs and correct the imbalance of yin and yang in the body.

"Nature" refers to the properties of the Chinese herbal medicines. Just like the different climates in four seasons, Chinese herbal medicines have four kinds of natures, including cold, hot, warm and cool. These four terms do not refer to the real temperature, but refer to the nature or property of the medicines. They are derived from the human body's response to the Chinese herbal medicines and the therapeutic effects of these medicines. For example, some diseases with heat syndromes need to be treated with medicines with cold nature, such as Juhua (chrysanthemum flower), Huanglian (rhizome of Chinese goldthread),

Baihe (lily bulb), Bohe (peppermint) and so on. These herbal medicines have the effects of clearing heat and toxicity and purging fire, etc. Some diseases with cold syndromes need to be treated with medicines with warm or hot nature, such as Renshen (ginseng), Danggui (Chinese angelica), Fangfeng (divaricate saposhnikovia root), etc. These medicines have the functions of warming spleen and stomach for dispelling cold and so on.

"Flavor" refers to the taste of drugs. "Five flavors" means the five basic flavors of Chinese medicines-pungent, sweet, sour, bitter and salty.

Pungent: The medicines with pungent flavor have the functions of volatilization, promoting the circulation of qi and invigorating the circulation of blood, etc. They are often used to treat exterior syndrome, such as Banxia (pinellia tuber), Zisu (perilla leaf), Baizhi (dahurian angelica root), Chuanxiong (Sichuan lovage rhizome), etc.

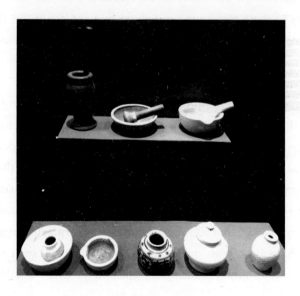

Sweet: The medicines with sweet flavor have the functions of regulating spleen and stomach, tonifying qi and blood, and alleviating pain, and they are suitable for the patients with deficient syndromes, and also can harmonize the properties of other medicines, such as Renshen (ginseng), Dangshen (tangshen), Gancao (liquorice root), Gouqizi (wolfberry fruit), etc.

Sour: The medicines with sour flavor have the functions of inducing astringency. They are often used to treat hyperhidrosis, diarrhea, spermatorrhea, urinary incontinence and so on, such as Wuweizi (Chinese Magnoliavine fruit), Shanzha (hawthorn fruit), Jinyingzi (Cherokee rose fruit), Fupenzi (palmleaf raspberry fruit) and so on.

Bitter: The medicines with bitter flavor have the functions of clearing heat and toxicity, drying dampness, reducing fire and purging stool, and are suitable for heat syndrome, damp-heat, carbuncle, sore, and ulcer, etc, such as Huanglian (rhizome of Chinese goldthread), Dahuang (rhubarb root and rhizome), Kuxingren (bitter apricot seed), etc.

Salty: The medcines with salty flavor have the functions of softening hardness to dissipate stagnation and defecation, etc, such as Wugong (centipede), Muli (oyster shell), Mangxiao (crystallized sodium sulfate) and so on.

四、中药的炮制 / Processing of Chinese herbal medicine

中药材采集后不能直接入药，要去除杂质或者非药用部位。某些具有毒性或者刺激性的药材，还需要通过炮制加以减缓。什么是中药炮制呢？简单地说，中药炮制就是根据用药需要和药物性质，对原药材进行一定的加工处理，以充分发挥中药的疗效，避免或减少一些不良反应，或改变中药原有的药性以更好地适应病情需要。

具体来说，中药炮制的目的主要有四个：

（一）增强中药的临床疗效

中药炮制往往需要增加一些辅料，如黄酒、蜂蜜、姜汁等等。这些辅料可以增强中药的疗效，如蜜炙甘草可以增强甘草的润肺止咳作用，盐炙杜仲可以增强杜仲的补肝肾作用。

（二）降低或消除药物的毒副作用，保证用药安全

一些中药是有毒的，这些中药如果口服使用，就必须经过炮制来消除或降低药物的毒性。比如川乌通过炮制可以大大减少有毒成分乌头碱的含量。陈皮需要陈制至少一年来减少陈皮中挥发油的含量。

（三）改变药物的性能或功效，以适应病情的需要

比如地黄本身性味甘寒，适宜清热凉血，但通过黄酒反复蒸制晾晒后变为熟地黄，药性由寒变温，用于补益精血。再如麻黄善于发汗解表，而用蜂蜜炒过后的蜜炙麻黄则增强了平喘止咳的功能。

（四）便于储存

刚采集的鲜药材含有大量水分，容易霉变，所以中药材在储存、运输等过程中必须要通过自然晾晒或烘干进行干燥处理。有些药材需要在产地进行盐处理以防霉变，如全蝎等。

中药的炮制大体包括如下方法：

1. 修制：对药材进行净化、粉碎或切制。属于药材的初加工，为后续进一步加工、调剂和临床用药做准备。如枇杷叶表面毛茸多，需刮去粗毛；皮类药材需要刮去粗皮；贝壳类药材需要进行粉碎；根类药材需要切片。

2. 水制：用水或其他液体辅料处理药材，主要是为了清洁、除杂、软化药材等目的。常见方法如漂洗、闷润、浸泡、喷洒、水飞等。

3. 火制：用火加工处理中药材。主要方式有炒、炙、烫、煅、煨、炮、燎、烘等。

4. 水火共制：主要有蒸法和煮法。如酒蒸地黄增加补肝肾和补血作用。

After collecting, the Chinese medicinal materials cannot be directly used. Impurities or non-medicinal parts should be removed. Some toxic or irritating medicines need to be processed through "processing". What is the processing of traditional Chinese medicine? In brief, it means to process the original medicinal materials according to the needs of medication and the nature of medicines, so as to give full play to the efficacy of traditional Chinese medicines, avoid or reduce some adverse reactions, or change the original medicinal properties to better meet the needs of diseases.

Specifically, there are four main purposes for the processing of traditional Chinese medicine:

1. Enhancing the clinical efficacy of traditional Chinese medicine

Some pharmaceutical excipients, such as rice wine, honey, ginger juice, are often used in the processing. They can enhance the efficacy of traditional Chinese medicine. For example, honey-roasted Gancao (liquorice root) can have better lung-moistening and cough-relieving effects. Salt-roasted Duzhong (eeucommia bark) will have better liver and Kidney-tonifying effects.

2. Reducing or eliminating toxic and side effects of herbal medicines to ensure medication safety

Some herbal medicines are toxic, and must be processed if they are used orally in order to reduce their toxicity. For example, aconitine in Chuanwu (common monkshood mother root) can be greatly reduced after processing. Chenpi (dried tangerine peel) needs to be aged for at least one year so that volatile oil in it can be reduced during aging.

3. Changing the performance or efficacy of herbal medicines to meet the needs of diseases

Dihuang (rehmannia root) is sweet and cold in nature. It is suitable for clearing heat and cooling blood. However, it changes to Shudihuang (prepared rehmannia root) after repeated steaming and drying with rice wine. Its medicinal properties change from cold to warm, and it is often used to tonify the blood. Besides, Mahuang (ephedra herb) is good at sweating and releasing exterior, while honey-fried Mahuang has better function of relieving asthma and cough.

4. Easy storage

Due to high moisture content, the freshly collected medicinal materials are easy to mildew. Therefore, they must be dried during storage and transportation, either through natural drying or oven drying. Some medicinal materials such as Quanxie (scorpion) need to be treated with salt in the producing area to prevent mildew.

The following methods are often used in processing of traditional Chinese medicine:

1. Preliminary processing: Including cleansing, crushing or cutting of medicinal materials. The preliminary processing of medicinal materials prepares for further processing, dispensing and clinical medication. For

example, loquat leaves are hairy and the thick hairs need to be scraped off; the rough barks of bark medicinal materials need to be scraped off; the shellfish medicinal materials need to be crushed; the root medicinal materials need to be sliced.

2. Processed with water: The processing of medicinal materials with water or other liquid excipients is mainly for cleaning, removing impurities and softening medicinal materials. Common methods include rinsing, moistening, soaking, spraying, grinding in water, etc.

3. Processed with fire: Some Chinese medicinal materials are processed by fire. The major methods include stir-frying, roasting, scalding, calcining, burning, baking, etc.

4. Co-processing with both water and fire: Mainly including steaming and boiling. For example, steaming Dihuang with wine can increase the liver-and-kidney-tonifying and blood-tonifying effects.

五、中药的配伍 / Concerted application of Chinese herbal medicine

中药的配伍应用是中医用药的主要形式。我们看到大夫给病人开的中药处方里的中药往往都存在一定的配伍关系。中药间配伍关系古人总结为"七情"，即"单行、相须、相使、相杀、相畏、相恶、相反"。除单行外，其余六种都是谈的中药间配伍关系。

所谓"单行"就是指用单味药治病，适用于病情单纯的情况，如独参汤就只有一味人参，常用于大补元气。但由于病情多复杂，单行药往往难以兼顾治疗，需要同时使用至少两种以上药物配伍使用才能治疗病症。七情中的"相须、相使"可以实现药物配伍后增强疗效，比如杏仁搭配甘草能够增强祛痰止咳的功效。"相杀、相畏"的配伍可以减轻或消除药物的毒副作用或烈性，比如生姜能减轻或消除生半夏的毒性。而"相恶、相反"的配伍会降低药物疗效或增加药物毒副作用，在中药配伍时要加以避免，比如藜芦能削弱人参的补气作用。

The concerted application is one of the main features of traditional Chinese medicine. It is often seen that there is a certain concerted relationship between the ingredients in Chinese medicines prescribed by the doctors. The concerted relationship between traditional Chinese medicines was summarized by our ancestors as "seven relations" including "drug used singly, mutual promotion, mutual enhancement, counteract toxicity of another drug, incompatibility, mutual inhibition, antagonism". Except for "drug used singly", the other six are all about concerted application of Chinese medicines.

The so-called "drug used singly" refers to the treatment of disease with only one single drug, which is suitable for simple conditions. For example, Dushen Decoction with Renshen (ginseng) as the main ingredient is often used to treat vitality deficiency. However, due to the complexity of diseases, it is often difficult to treat diseases with only one herbal medicine. Instead, it is necessary to use at least two or more herbal medicines at the same time. "Mutual promotion" and "mutual enhancement" mean the efficacy of some herbal medicines can be enhanced when concerted applied. For example, almond used with licorice will have better expectorant and cough reliving effects. The application of "counteract toxicity of another drug" and "incompatibility" can alleviate or eliminate the toxic side effects or intensity of drugs. For instance, ginger can alleviate or eliminate the toxicity of raw Banxia (pinellia tuber). However, the application based on "mutual inhibition" and "antagonism" will reduce the efficacy or increase the toxicity and side effects of some herbal medicines, which should be avoided in the application of traditional Chinese medicine. For example, Lilu (falsehellebore root and rhizome) can weaken the tonifying effect of Renshen (ginseng).

六、中药的煎制 / Decoction of Chinese herbal medicine

中药的煎制有一定的要求，但只要掌握好正确的方法就很简单。

（一）煎药工具

煎煮中药最好用砂锅、陶器和瓦罐等，也可用搪瓷器皿或不锈钢锅。切忌用铁、铝、锡和铜等金属容器，因为金属容易和中药产生化学反应而影响药效。

（二）煎药过程

煎药可以用自来水或是凉开水。中药一般要煎两次。首次煎煮（一煎）前将一剂中药饮片材料放入煲内，加入清水没过药物2至3厘米，一般药物浸泡30分钟，可以帮助有效成分煎出，浸泡药材的水不用倒掉，直接和药材一起煮，先用大火煎沸，然后改用小火再煎20～30分钟，之后滤取药液。再次煎煮（二煎）时，不用再浸泡，加水淹没药物即可，依上法煎煮，取第二次药液。将两次药液混匀，遵医嘱服用。

（三）煎药时间

煎煮的时间都是从药液煮沸后开始计算。解表类药（比如治感冒的药物）：头煎需10～15分钟，二煎需10分钟左右。一般类药（比如治咳嗽的药物）：头煎需20～25分钟，二煎需15～20分钟。滋补类药（如调理的药物）：头煎需40～50分钟，二煎需25～30分钟。

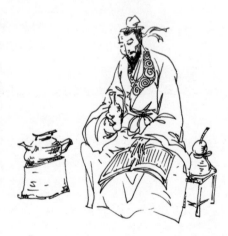

（四）特殊药物

还有一些药物需要用特殊的方法来煎煮，这些药物通常会单独包装。

"先煎药"：一般是矿物、贝壳类、角甲类或有毒性的药物，如石膏、牡蛎、龟甲和附子等，需要先用少量水煮沸10～15分钟，然后再与其他药同煎。

"后下药"：一般是含有挥发油的药物，如薄荷、紫苏和广藿香等，在头煎结束前的五分钟时，放入药锅内同煎5分钟即可。

"包煎药"：有些药材质地极细或过轻，煎煮时容易漂浮在药液面上，有些药材含淀粉、黏液质较多，煎煮时容易粘锅、糊化，有些药材有毛或杂质，容易刺激咽喉或消化道。如车前子、辛夷等，就需要用纱布包裹好再煎。

"烊化药"：烊化是指把胶类药物放入热溶液（如水、黄酒或煎好的药液）中溶化，再倒入药液中搅拌均匀服用，比如阿胶、鹿角胶等。

"冲服药"：一般是粉剂药物，如羚羊角粉，将药调入煎好的药汁或开水中冲服。

There are certain requirements for the decoction of Chinese medicine, but it would be very simple as long as you master the correct method.

(1) Decoction tools

It would be better to decoct Chinese herbal medicine in casserole, pottery, or crock pots, etc. Enamel or stainless steel pots are also acceptable. But never use iron, aluminum, tin, copper and other metal containers, because this will cause chemical reactions, and thus reduce the medical effects.

(2) Decoction process

Either tap water or cold boiled water is suitable for decoction. The medicine need to be decocted twice. Before the first decoction, put a dose of medicine into the pot, and then add water into the pot until the water is 2 to 3 centimeters higher than the medicine. Then let it soak for 30 minutes, because soaking can help get more effective ingredients from herbs during decoction. The water needn't be poured out. Firstly the intense fire is used until the water is boiled, and then let it simmer on slow fire for 20-30 minutes. The liquid is filtered. The next step is the second decoction. Water is added until it submerges the medicine, but there is no need for another soaking. Then following the procedure does in the first decoction. After getting the liquid, mix the two fluids and take them by following the doctor's advice.

(3) Decoction time

Decoction time is calculated after the water is boiled. The medicine for relieving the exterior syndrome (like medicine for cold): 10-15 minutes for the first decoction, and 10 minutes for the second decoction. The common medicine (like medicine for coughs): 20-25 minutes for the first decoction, and 15-20 minutes for the second decoction. Nourishing medicine (like medicine for conditioning human bodies): 40-50 minutes for the first decoction, and 25-30 minutes for the second decoction.

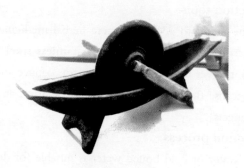

传统的药碾

(4) Special medicines

There are some medicines which need to be decocted in special ways. These medicines are usually packaged separately.

"Decocted earlier": Generally speaking, minerals, shells, horns or toxic medicines, such as Shigao (gypsum), Muli (oyster shell), Guijia (tortoise's carapace and plastron), Fuzi (prepared common monkshood branched root), etc., need to be boiled with a small amount of water for 10-15 minutes before the decoction, and then they can be decocted together with other herbs.

"Decocted later": Some herbs containing volatile oils, such as Bohe (peppermint), Zisu (perilla leaf), Guanghuoxiang (cablin potchouli herb), etc., can be put in the pot five minutes before the end of the first decoction and decocted for 5 minutes.

"Wrapped medicine": Some medicines are too fine or light, and they are likely to float on the surface of the liquid during decoction; some medicines contain much starch or mucus, and they are easy to stick to the pot or even cause gelatinization; some medicines have hairs or impurities, which can easily irritate the throat or digestive tract. These medicines such as Cheqianzi (plantain seed) and Xinyi (biond magnolia flower-bud) need to be wrapped with gauze during decoction.

"Melting method": This method means to melt some kinds of gelatin medicines in hot liquid (such as water, rice wine or decocted liquid), and then the melted medicines are mixed with the decocted liquid for people to take. Such drugs include Ejiao (donkey hide gelatin) or Lujiaojiao (deer-horn glue), etc.

"Mixing method": Generally, some kinds of powder medicines, such as Lingyangjiao Fen (powder of antelope horn), need be mixed in the decoction or boiled water for people to take.

七、中药的服用和禁忌 /
Usage and contraindications of Chinese herbal medicine

一般来说，一剂药分两次服用，一般在饭后服为宜，需要和吃饭错开半小时左右。但不同药物有不同的要求，具体时间如下。

宜饭前服用的中药：①补益药，饭前服用利于吸收；②制酸止痛类胃病药物，饭前服用可以增强对胃黏膜的保护；③祛痰止咳平喘药，宜饭前服用；④驱虫药，宜空腹服用，利于驱虫。

宜饭后服用的中药：①解表药最好在中午饭后服用；②健胃药最好在饭后片刻服用，以达到消食化积的作用；③辛辣刺激性药物宜在饭后服用，以防止刺激胃黏膜。

宜睡前服用的中药：①安神药应在睡前1小时左右服用，有利患者入睡；②润肠通便药，应睡前服用，有利于消除胃肠积滞。

此外，服用中药时也有一些注意事项，如下。

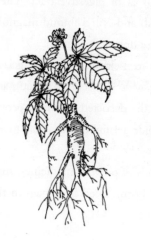

（1）服中药时忌生、冷和油腻的食物。

（2）服中药时不要喝浓茶。

（3）服中药时不能吃辣椒，特别是热性的病症。

（4）服用人参、党参期间，忌食生萝卜、绿豆。

（5）消化不良者，忌食油炸黏腻不易消化的食物。

（6）疮疡脓肿等病忌食鱼、虾、蟹等腥膻食物。

Generally speaking, one dose of medicine is taken twice a day, usually half an hour after meals. However, different kinds of medicine should be taken at different time, and the specific time for taking medicine is as follows.

The medicine taken before meals: (1) tonic medicine is taken before meal, which is conducive to absorption; (2) the medicine which inhibits gastric acid is usually taken before meals as this can protect gastric mucosa; (3) the medicine which aims to dispel phlegm and relieve coughing is also taken before meals; (4) deworming medicine should also be taken on an empty stomach, which can help repel worms.

The medicine taken after meals: (1) the medicine for relieving exterior disorder is best taken after lunch; (2) that for stomachic tonic is best taken after meals since it can help digestion; (3) some pungent or stimulant medicine should be taken after meals to prevent irritation of gastric mucosa.

The medicine taken before bed time: (1) tranquilizing medicine should be taken about an hour before going to bed, which can help patients fall asleep; (2) the medicine relaxing the bowels should be taken before going to bed, which is conducive to eliminating gastrointestinal stagnation.

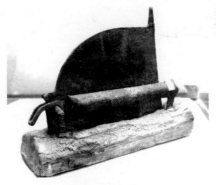

传统的中药切药刀

Besides, there are also some contraindications when taking Chinese medicine, such as:

(1) People should avoid raw, cold and greasy food while taking Chinese herbal medicine;

(2) People should not drink strong tea while taking Chinese herbal medicine;

(3) People should not eat chilies, especially the patients with heat syndrome;

(4) When taking Renshen (ginseng) and Dangshen (tangshen), people should avoid raw radish or mung bean;

(5) People with indigestion should avoid fried foods or sticky foods as they are not easy to digest;

(6) People with some problems such as sores or abscess should avoid fishy food such as fish, shrimp, crab and so on.

第二章　五十种常见中药介绍

An introduction to fifty common Chinese herbal medicines

本章着重介绍五十种常见和常用的中药，希望能帮助读者朋友们对它们有一个初步的认识。每种中药的介绍包括知识模块、拓展模块和故事模块。知识模块包括中药的来源、产地、本草始载、功效和主治；拓展模块对这些中药在其他方面的应用进行了简介，如食品、养生、美容和绿化等方面；故事模块中，我们搜集整理了与这些中药有关的民间传说、奇闻逸事和历史故事等，这些故事生动有趣，能进一步加深我们对这些中药的理解。

　　按照中药的来源，本章中的这五十种中药分为植物类、真菌类、动物类和矿物类四大类，其中植物类药又根据药用部位做了进一步的细分。为了体现出中国文化的特色，每一类里的中药是按照笔画进行的排序。

　　另外，需要注意的是，拉丁语是许多学科的国际通用语言，尤其是医药学、动植物学和微生物学等学科的命名和术语，均使用拉丁语，以避免语言不同而产生的混乱和误解。每味中药也有它的拉丁名，有利于国际的交流、贸易和合作研究。在本书中所提到的动植物的名称及其科属均提供了相对应的拉丁学名，每种中药的汉语名称的后面均提供了汉语拼音、英文名和拉丁名（本书中的药材拉丁名参考了中医药学名词审定委员会《中医药学术语》第一版）。同时，在英文段落中，当涉及中药名称的时候，大多都使用了汉语拼音，这样能使外国读者对中国文化能有更好的了解。

This chapter focuses on the introduction of 50 commonly seen and commonly used Chinese herbal medicines, hoping to help readers have a preliminary understanding of them. The introduction of each medicine includes Basic Knowledge, Related Information and Story. Basic Knowledge includes their origin, location, in which books they are first recorded, efficacy and indications; Related Information introduces the application of these Chinese herbal medicines in other aspects, such as food, health, beauty products, greening and so on; in Story part, we have collected some vivid and interesting folklores, anecdotes, and historical stories related to these Chinese herbal medicines in order to deepen readers' understanding of them.

According to their sources, these 50 kinds of Chinese herbal medicine in this chapter can be divided into four categories: botanical, fungus, animal and mineral medicines. The botanical medicines are further divided according to the medicinal parts. In order to emphasize the Chinese culture, these Chinese herbal medicines in each category are sorted according to the strokes of their Chinese names.

In addition, it should be noted that Latin is the international language of many disciplines, such as medical science, zoology, plant science, microbiology, etc. Latin is used in the naming and terminology of these disciplines in order to avoid confusion and misunderstanding caused by different languages. Therefore, each Chinese medicine has its Latin name, which is conducive to international communication, trade and cooperative research. The names of animals and plants and their families and genera in this book all have corresponding scientific names in Latin (these Latin names come from *Terminology of Traditional Chinese Medicine* compiled by Committee for Terms in Traditional Chinese Medicine). The Chinese names of medicines in this book are followed by their Chinese Pinyin, English names and Latin names. At the same time, when it comes to the names of medicines in the English paragraphs, their Chinese Pinyin will be used so that foreign readers can have a better understanding of Chinese culture.

一、植物类 / Botanical medicine

植物类中药占所有中药的绝大部分,大概占到整个中药的90%左右,所以"中药"在古代叫作"本草"。根据植物部位不同,植物类中药分为如下几种。

根和根茎类:根和根茎是植物类中药最重要的入药部位。这里的根茎类泛指植物地下变态茎,包括根茎、块茎、鳞茎和球茎。

全草类:主要指草本植物的地上部分。

花类:指植物的花蕾、盛开的花、花序或者花的某一部分(如花粉、雌蕊柱头等)。

果实种子类:主要指入药的植物果实或者种子。

皮类:主要指植物的茎皮和枝皮。根皮类中药一般归到根和根茎类药材中。

茎木类:包括茎类中药和木类中药。茎类中药常指木本植物的茎,以及少数草本植物的茎藤;木类中药指木本植物的木质茎,常以心材(即树木中心部位的木材)为主要来源。

树脂类:植物分泌的树脂,如乳香、没药和血竭。

其他类:指植物某一部分加工品,如芦荟;蕨类植物孢子,如海金沙;植物分泌的非树脂类物质,如天竺黄。

藻、菌和地衣类:此类中药较为低等。除藻类属于低等植物外,菌类(真菌)和地衣类并不属于植物。传统分类方法把它们并入植物中的藻、菌和地衣类处理。本书为了突出生物的自然属性,未把常见的真菌类药材归入植物类药,而是单独处理。

Botanical Chinese medicines account for the vast majority (about 90%) of all Chinese medicines, so "Chinese medicine" in ancient times was called "Ben Cao" (herbal medicine). According to the different parts of plants, botanical medicines can be divided into the following categories.

Root and rhizome: Roots and rhizomes are the most important part of Chinese herbal medicines. Rhizome here generally refers to underground modified stems of plants, including rhizomes, tubers, bulbs and corms.

Whole herb: It mainly refers to the aboveground parts of herbaceous plants.

Flower: It refers to buds, blooming flowers, inflorescences, or other parts of flowers (such as pollen, pistil stigma, etc).

Fruit and seed: Fruit and seed mainly refer to the fruits or seeds of plants that are used as medicines.

Bark: It mainly refers to the stem bark and branch bark of plants. Root bark is generally classified into Root and Rhizome category.

Stem and wood: They include stem medicine and wood medicine. Stem medicine refers to the stem of woody plants and also the stems and vines of some herbaceous plants. Wood medicine refers to the woody stem of plants, often from heartwood (i.e. the wood in the center of the tree).

Resin: Resin is secreted by plants, such as Ruxiang (frankincense), Moyao (myrrh), Xuejie (draconis resin).

Others: They are processed products of certain part of the plant, such as Luhui (aloe); spores of ferns, such as Haijinsha (Japanese climbing fern spore); non-resinous substance secreted by plant, such as Tianzhuhuang (tabasheer).

Alga, fungus and lichens: These kinds of Chinese medicines are relatively lower. Alga is a kind of lower plant, while fungi and lichens are not plants. According to traditional classification methods, alga medicine, fungus medicine and lichen medicine all belong to botanical medicine. However, in order to highlight the natural attributes of fungus medicine, the fungus medicine will be discussed later in another part, instead of being included in botanical medicine.

（一）根和根茎类 / Root and rhizome

人参
Renshen / Ginseng / Radix Ginseng

知识模块

来源： 五加科（Araliaceae）植物人参 *Panax ginseng* C. A. Mey. 的干燥根及根茎。

产地： 主产于吉林、辽宁等省。栽培的称为园参，野生的称为山参，种于林下自然生长的称为林下参。

本草始载： 始载于东汉《神农本草经》。

功效： 大补元气，补脾益肺，生津，安神。

主治： 治疗各种气虚导致的疾病，为重要的滋补类中药。

Basic knowledge

Origin: The dry root and rhizome of *Panax ginseng* C. A. Mey. belong to the family Araliaceae.

Location: Renshen is mainly produced in Jilin and Liaoning provinces, etc. The artificially cultivates ones are called as Yuan Shen (garden Renshen), the wild ones are called as Shan Shen (mountain Renshen), and those grown in the forest are called as Lin Xia Shen (Renshen in forest).

First recorded in: *Shennong's Classic of Materia Medica* of the Eastern Han Dynasty.

Efficacy: Tonifying primordial qi, invigorating spleen for benefiting lung, promoting the production of body fluid, and inducing tranquilization.

Indications: Renshen can treat various diseases caused by qi deficiency. Renshen is an important nourishing medicine.

拓展模块

人参是我国著名的中药材，中国古代称它为"百草之王"和"神草"，是闻名遐迩的"东北三宝"（人参、貂皮和鹿茸）之一。人参（地下部分）形态似人形，有脖子、脑袋和胳膊腿儿，故名"人参"，谐音"人身"。

由于人参具有很好的滋补强壮的功能，是一种非常好的保健品，一直以来受到国人的推崇。人参的吃法也很多，可以用水煮着吃、蒸着吃，或是泡水或泡酒喝，也可以用来做粥或炖汤，如常见的人参鸡汤不仅做法简单，而且是一道滋补佳品，具有补脾益肺、安神定志和补气生血等功效。

人参大补元气，一般人群均可食用，尤适宜身体虚弱者、气血不足者、气短者、贫血者和神经衰弱者。但是，有实证、热证的人不宜服用人参，如感冒发热、气喘、咽喉肿痛和失眠多梦等症，而且怀孕后期的女性也不宜服用人参。同时，需要注意人参不可与含鞣酸的水果，如葡萄以及生萝卜、海鲜和茶叶等同服。

Related information

Renshen is a famous herbal medicine in China. In the ancient times, it was called "king of herbs" and "magical herb". It is one of the famous "three treasures of Northeast China" (Renshen, mink fur and Lurong/velvet antler). The underground part of Renshen looks like the human body, which has a neck, a head, arms and legs, hence the name Renshen (which has the same pronunciation of "人身", the Chinese name of human body).

Renshen with good nourishing and strengthening effects is a very good health food, so it has always been popular among Chinese people. Renshen can be boiled, steamed, and soaked in water or wine before being taken. It can also be used to make porridge or soup. For example, Renshen-chicken soup is not only simple to cook, but also a good nourishing food. It has the functions of invigorating spleen and lung, calming mind, invigorating qi and blood, etc.

Renshen is good for invigorating vital energy and can be taken by the common people, especially for those with poor health, qi and blood deficiency, shortness of breath, anemia and neurasthenia. However, the people with excess syndrome or heat syndrome should not take Renshen, such as cold accompanied with fever, asthma, sore throat, insomnia and dreaminess, and women in the late pregnancy should not take it either. At the same time, it should be noted that Renshen had better not be taken together with tannin-rich fruits such as grapes, as well as raw radish, seafood and tea, etc.

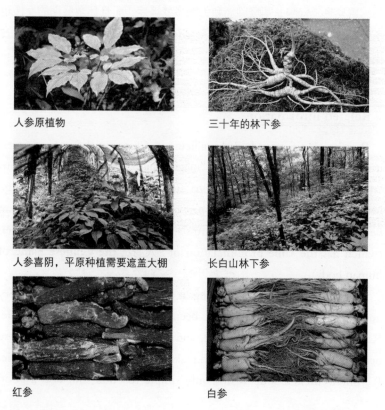

人参原植物　　　　　　　　　三十年的林下参

人参喜阴，平原种植需要遮盖大棚　　长白山林下参

红参　　　　　　　　　　　　白参

故事模块

　　相传很久以前，在沂蒙山上生长着许多人参，其中两棵活了上千年，有了灵性，化身成为两个可爱的人参娃娃。

　　一天，一个黑心和尚带着清风、明月两个小徒弟来到山上。每天晚上这个黑心和尚就在山上到处寻找人参娃娃。两个小和尚整天干活，还经常挨打受骂。机缘巧合之下，两个人参娃娃和清风、明月成了好朋友，但这件事被黑心和尚发现了。他就哄骗清风、明月把一根红线偷偷拴到人参娃娃的身上。随后，黑心和尚顺着红线，果然在大山深处找到了人参娃娃，并带回来放进锅里准备煮熟吃掉。幸好被清风、明月及时发现，他俩不顾一切把人参娃娃救了出来，让他们从后院逃走。

　　逃出虎口的人参娃娃带着他们的家族，迁到了我国东北的大森林里，在那里安家落户，繁衍生息。至于那个狠心的坏和尚也得到了应有的惩罚。

　　虽然这只是一个虚构的传说故事，为人参蒙上了一层神秘的面纱，但也让人们了解道，我们要珍惜大自然的馈赠，不可大肆破坏和掠夺，要取之有度，才能用之不竭！

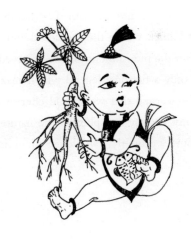

Story

According to legend, long time ago, there were many Renshen growing on the Yimeng Mountain of Shandong Province. Two of them lived for over a thousand years and turned into two adorable Renshen babies.

One day, an evil monk arrived in the mountain with two disciples-Qingfeng (which literally means "cool breeze") and Mingyue (which literally means "bright moon"). The evil monk looked for Renshen babies in the mountains every night. The two young monks worked all day but were still often abused by the evil monk. By accident, the two Renshen babies became good friends with Qingfeng and Mingyue. But this was discovered by the evil monk. He coaxed Qingfeng and Mingyue into tying a red thread onto the babies. Later, the evil monk found two Renshen babies with the help of the red thread and took them back. He put the Renshen babies in a pot and tried to cook them. Fortunately, this was found by Qingfeng and Mingyue in time. They rescued the Renshen babies and helped them to escape from the backyard.

The Renshen babies then moved with their family to the big forest in the Northeast of China, where they settled down and thrived. And the evil monk also got the punishment that he deserved.

Although this is only a fictional legend which makes Renshen very mysterious, it can be learned that we should cherish the gift given by nature, and should not destroy and plunder the nature. Only when we take the natural resources properly, can we use them inexhaustibly.

大黄

Dahuang / Rhubarb Root and Rhizome / Radix et Rhizoma Rhei

知识模块

来源：蓼科（Polygonaceae）植物掌叶大黄 *Rheum palmatum* L.、唐古特大黄 *R. tanguticum* Maxim. ex Balf. 或药用大黄 *R. officinale* Baill. 的干燥根和根茎。

产地：产于青海、甘肃及西南等地。

本草始载：始载于东汉《神农本草经》。

功效：泻下通便，清热泻火，解毒，止血，活血祛瘀。

主治：常用于治疗大便秘结，热毒肿痛，血热出血等。

Basic knowledge

Origin: The dry root and rhizome of *Rheum palmatum* L., *R. tanguticum* Maxim. ex Balf. or *R. officinale* Baill. belonging to the family Polygonaceae.

Location: Dahuang is mainly produced in Qinghai Province, Gansu Province and Southwestern China.

First recorded in: *Shennong's Classic of Materia Medica* of the Eastern Han Dynasty.

Efficacy: Relaxing the bowels with purgation, clearing heat-fire, removing toxicity, stopping bleeding, activating blood and dispelling stasis.

Indications: Constipation, sores and abscess due to heat-toxin, bleeding due to heat in blood.

拓展模块

大黄作为我国传统中药，很早就沿丝绸之路传入欧洲。据说，由于西方国家以牛羊肉及奶制品为主要食材，致使热性体征明显，容易产生便秘等疾病，一直无法很好解决，直到大黄出现在欧洲才得到解决，自此大黄被西方视为神物，有时甚至成为战争必夺之物。后来，欧洲人栽培出了可食用的大黄（*Rheum rhaponticum* L.），叶柄部分可供食用，用在馅饼、酥皮点心等甜食里，如大黄草莓派或大黄草莓酱。18世纪末，缅因州的一名菜农把大黄的种子由欧洲带到北美。

大黄有很高的药用价值，常用于实热便秘、湿热黄疸和咽喉肿痛等，但脾胃虚寒、气血虚弱者及产后、哺乳期女性均慎服，孕妇禁服。

Related information

As a Chinese herbal medicine, Dahuang was introduced to Europe very early through the Silk Road. It is said that people in Western countries took the beef, mutton and milk products as the main ingredients of their everyday food, resulting in obvious symptoms of heat syndrome. So relevant diseases such as constipation prevailed, and could not be cured for quite a long time. The situation lasted until the emergence of Dahuang. So Dahuang was considered to be divine in the Western world, and was sometimes even the cause of wars. Later, the people in Europe cultivated edible Dahuang-rhubarb (*Rheum rhaponticum* L.) whose petiole can be eaten. It can be made into pies and desserts, such as rhubarb strawberry pie or rhubarb strawberry sauce. At the end of the 18th century, a vegetable farmer in Maine, USA brought its seeds from Europe to North America.

Dahuang has a high medicinal value. It is often used to treat constipation of excess heat type, damp-heat jaundice, and sore throat and so on. However, the people with the deficiency-cold in spleen and stomach, qi and blood deficiency, as well as postpartum and lactating women should be cautious when taking it. And it is forbidden for pregnant women.

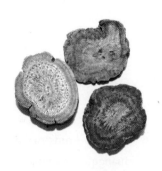 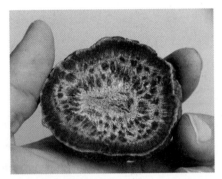

大黄根茎断面可见"星点"

故事模块

　　相传从前有一位郎中，善于用黄连、黄芪、黄精、黄芩和黄根这五味药材给人治病，人称"五黄先生"。

　　五黄先生收了个徒弟名叫马骏，让他跟着自己采药卖药，但却从不教他如何行医，因为他觉得马骏性子太急，不适合当郎中。马骏心有不满，就偷偷学了一些医术，背着五黄先生给人治病。机缘巧合，还真治好了几个人。

　　有一天，一位孕妇因为腹泻来找郎中，但五黄先生不在，马骏就擅自为病人开药。本来止泻应该用黄连，马骏却错给她用了泻火的黄根。病人吃过药后，大泻不止，没过两天就死了。愤怒的病人家属把马骏扭送进了县衙。五黄先生闻讯赶来，自请有罪："他是跟我学的医术，我没有教清楚，罪在我身。"马骏急忙说："老爷，是我背着五黄先生给人开药，跟他完全没关系。"县官问明情况后，罚他们赔偿给死者家里一大笔钱，这才算了事。马骏羞愧万分，从此踏踏实实，人也变得稳重多了，五黄先生这才教他行医。

为了记住这次的惨痛教训，五黄先生从此便将黄根这味药改名为"大黄"，强调它的功效之猛，免得后人错用。这个故事也告诉我们，如果医生疏忽大意给病人用错了药，可是会造成很严重的后果。其实无论从事什么职业，工作中都要细心严谨才行。

Story

According to the legend, once upon a time, there was a doctor who was good at treating people with five kinds of herbal medicines-Huanglian, Huangqi, Huangjing, Huangqin and Huanggen. So he was called "Mr. Wuhuang" (which literally means "five yellow").

Mr. Wuhuang had a student named Ma Jun, and he asked Ma Jun to collect and sell medicinal herbs with him but never taught him how to treat diseases, because he thought that Ma Jun was too short tempered to be a doctor. Dissatisfied, Ma Jun secretly learned some medical skills. When Mr. Wuhuang was absent from the clinic, Ma Jun would take his place to treat patients. Unexpectedly, he did cure several people.

One day, a pregnant woman came to the clinic because of diarrhea, but Mr. Wuhuang was absent, and thus Ma Jun prescribed some medicine for the woman. Diarrhea was supposed to be treated with Huanglian, but Ma Jun mistakenly gave her Huanggen. After the patient took the medicine, her diarrhea became more severe, and she died a couple of days later. The patient's family angrily sent Ma Jun to the magistrate's. Mr. Wuhuang heard the news and went to the magistrate's to plead guilty, "Ma Jun learned medical skills from me. I didn't teach him well, so I should take all the blame." Hearing this, Ma Jun said regretfully, "It was me who gave the prescription to the patient. He had nothing to do with this at all." After the county magistrate made clear the situation, Mr. Wuhuang and Ma were fined a large sum of money to compensate the family of the deceased woman. Ma Jun was ashamed, and since then he became more prudent and modest, therefore Mr. Wuhuang was finally determined to teach him how to treat diseases.

In order to remember the painful lesson, Mr. Wuhuang changed the name of Huanggen to "Dahuang" since then, emphasizing its strong effect, so that people in the future would not misuse this medicine. The story also tells us that it would cause serious consequences if doctors prescribed wrong medicines. Actually whatever jobs people do, they all should take the job patiently and seriously.

山药

Shanyao / Common Yam Rhizome / Rhizoma Dioscoreae

知识模块

来源： 薯蓣科（Dioscoreaceae）植物薯蓣 *Dioscorea opposita* Thunb. 的根茎。

产地： 主产于河南、河北。湖南、江西、广东和广西亦产。产于河南焦作的山药称为"怀山药"，河北安平、蠡县等地的山药称为"小白嘴山药"。

本草始载： 始载于东汉《神农本草经》。

功效： 益气养阴，补脾肺肾。

主治： 治疗脾虚证、肺虚证、肾虚证及消渴症等。

Basic knowledge

Origin: The rhizome of *Dioscorea opposita* Thunb. belonging to the family Diosoreaceae.

Location: Shanyao is mainly produced in Henan Province and Hebei Province. It is also produced in Hunan Province, Jiangxi Province, Guangdong Province, and Guangxi Province. Those produced in Henan are called "Huai Shanyao". Those produced in Anping County and Lixian County of Hebei Province are called "Xiaobaizui Shanyao" (which literally means "small white mouth Shanyao").

First recorded in: *Shennong's Classic of Materia Medica* of the Eastern Han Dynasty.

Efficacy: Benefiting qi and nourishing yin, tonifying spleen, lung and kidney.

Indications: Spleen deficiency syndrome, lung deficiency syndrome, kidney deficiency syndrome, diabetes.

山药营养价值丰富，而且物美价廉，是一味药食两用佳品，收载于原卫生部（现为中华人民共和国国家卫生健康委员会）发布的《既是食品又是药品的物品名单》。它有利于脾胃消化吸收功能，临床上常用来治脾胃虚弱、食少体倦、泄泻等病症。山药的道地药材是怀山药，产于河南焦作（原怀庆府）。怀山药中比较常见的一种是铁棍山药，因它的表面有像铁锈一样的痕迹，故得名铁棍山药。

山药有很多做法，可以蒸着吃、炒着吃，也可以煮粥或炖汤，像山药排骨汤、山药羊肉汤都是美味又滋补的佳品，还有甜点拔丝山药和蓝莓山药也非常受人们的喜爱。但是在削山药皮时如果直接用手接触到黏液，会导致手痒，这是因为山药皮里含皂角素，黏液里含生物碱。所以可以在削皮时戴上手套，或是手痒的话可用醋洗手加以缓解。

Related information

Shanyao, with various nutrients and a low price, can be used as both food and medicine, and has been included in *List of Items That Are both Food* and Medicine issued by former Ministry of Health(Now the National Health Commission,PRC). Beneficial for digestion and absorption functions of the spleen and stomach, it is commonly used in clinic to treat spleen deficiency, lack of appetite, body fatigue, and diarrhea and so on. The Huai Shanyao produced in Jiaozuo (formerly known as Huaiqingfu) of Henan Province is thought to be the best. And the most common type of Huai Shanyao is called Tiegun Shanyao because the spots on the surface are like iron rust (Tiegun means an iron bar).

Shanyao can be steamed, stir fried, cooked in porridge or stewed in soups. Shanyao-sparerib soup and Shanyao-mutton soup are both delicious and nourishing. Besides, desserts such as Ba Si Shanyao (Chinese yam in hot toffee) and Lan Mei Shanyao (Chinese yam with blueberry sauce) are also very popular. But when peeling Shanyao, if you touch its mucus directly with hands, You hands will be itchy, because Shanyao contains saponin, and its mucus contains alkaloids. So you can wear gloves when peeling Shanyao, or wash your hands with vinegar if they are itchy.

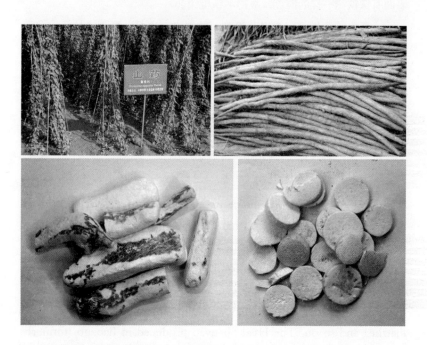

故事模块

战国时期，列国混战。有个强国把一个弱国打败了，弱国只剩下了几千人马，逃进一座大山中。强国的军队把大山包围，想把对方困死山中。谁知这样过了一年，山里连一点动静也没有。强国的官兵都认为山里的人马早就饿死了。

可是，忽然在一天夜里，从山中杀出一支人强马壮的队伍，直向强国的大营冲来。强国被杀了一个措手不及。结果，强国反败为胜，把失去的土地又夺了回来。

强国失败后很是奇怪，便四处探听弱国军队被困在山里时拿什么当粮食。后来才得知，原来山中到处都长着一种植物，它的根茎很粗。弱国的士兵饿急了，就挖这种根茎吃。从此，人吃根茎，马吃藤叶，几千人马靠这种植物生活了一年。弱国的士兵还给它起了个名字，叫"山遇"。意思是说碰巧在山里遇上了它。

后来人们发现，这种"山遇"不但营养丰富，还能够健脾胃，补肺肾，主治脾虚、泄泻等症。以后，人们用它做药，就把"山遇"这个名字改成"山药"了。

当然这只是个传说故事，事实上山药在古代被称为薯蓣，唐朝时，唐代宗名叫李豫，薯蓣跟皇帝同名怎么行呢，因此为了避讳，薯蓣就被改为了薯药，后来在北宋时因宋英宗名叫赵曙，薯药又为了避讳而被更名为山药，这个名字一直沿用至今。

Story

During the Warring States period, the states fought each other. A powerful state defeated a weak one. The weak state had only a few thousand people left and they fled into a mountain. The army of the powerful state besieged the mountain, hoping to trap the army of the weak state in the mountain until they were starved to death or forced to surrender. Nearly a year passed, the powerful army heard nothing from the mountain. So they believed that the people in the mountains had already starved to death.

However, one night, from the mountains, a bunch of strong men on strong horses suddenly rushed to the military camp of the powerful state. The army of the powerful state had no preparation for battle, so the weak state won the battle and recaptured their land.

After the failure, people in the powerful state were puzzled. They wondered what the weak army ate when they were blocked in the mountain. Later, they learned that there was a plant with thick roots all over in the mountains. Soldiers from the weak state had nothing to eat. They were so hungry that they began to dig the roots of this strange plant to feed their stomach. Since then, soldiers ate the roots and horses fed on its leaves. Thousands of people lived on this plant for almost a year. The soldiers gave it the name "Shan Yu" which literally means "encountering it in the mountain".

Later, people found that the root of the plant was not only nutritious, but also able to strengthen the spleen and stomach, supplement the lung and kidney, attending spleen deficiency, diarrhea and other symptoms. Later, when people used it as a medicine, they changed its name from "Shan Yu" to "Shan Yao" ("Shan" means "mountain" and "Yao" means "medicine").

Of course, this is only a legendary story. In fact, Shanyao was called Shuyu in ancient times. In Tang Dynasty, the name of Emperor Daizong was Li Yu, and it was a taboo to have the same or similar name with the emperors, so Shuyu was changed to Shuyao. Later in Northern Song Dynasty, the name of Emperor Yingzong was Zhao Shu, so Shuyao was then changed into Shanyao, which is still used today.

川乌

Chuanwu / Common Monkshood Mother Root / Radix Aconiti

知识模块

来源：毛茛科（Ranunculaceae）植物乌头 *Aconitum carmichaeli* Debx. 的干燥母根。

产地：产于四川、陕西等地。

本草始载：始载于唐代《药谱》。

功效：祛风胜湿，温经止痛。

主治：常用于治疗关节肿痛，风寒湿痹。

Basic knowledge

Origin: The dry tuberous root of *Aconitum carmichaeli* Debx. belonging to the family Ranunculaceae.

Location: Chuanwu is mainly produced in Sichuan and Shaanxi provinces.

First recorded in: *Yao Pu* (*Pedigree of Medicinal Herbs*) of the Tang Dynasty.

Efficacy: Dispelling wind-damp, warming meridians and alleviating pain.

Indications: Joint swelling and pain, wind-cold-dampness arthralgia.

拓展模块

川乌也叫乌头，你知道这个名字的由来吗？陶弘景描述它为"春时茎初生有脑头，形如乌鸟之头，故谓之乌头"，就是说川乌的块根形态上像一个乌鸦的脑袋。你们看图片里的川乌根像吗？它的子根叫作附子，功效主治与乌头相似。需要注意的是，川乌含有乌头碱，有大毒，被载入《保健食品禁用物品名单》。川乌必须经过炮制后方可使用，口服的话需要久煎，并且孕妇忌用。

Related information

Chuanwu is also called Wutou (which literally means the head of a crow). Do you know why? Tao Hongjing described it in this way "when the root of the herb begins to grow in the spring, it looks like the head of a crow". Look at the following picture, do you think so? The secondary root of the plant is named Fuzi (prepared common monkshood branched root), which has similar effects with Chuanwu. What's important is that Chuanwu contains aconitine which is highly toxic, and thus it is included in the List of Items That Are Prohibited in Health Food. Therefore, it must be processed before being used. It needs to be decocted for a long time when taken internally, and it mustn't be taken by pregnant women.

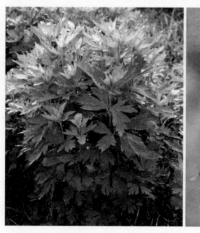
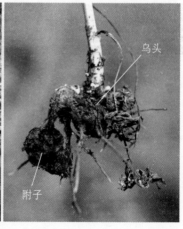

乌头

附子

大家肯定听过《三国演义》中华佗为关羽"刮骨疗毒"的故事，说的是关羽在攻打樊城时，右臂中了毒箭。华佗检查后发现关羽是被乌头的毒所伤，需要刮去骨头上的毒素。在征得关羽同意后，华佗开始为他进行手术。华佗在关羽的右胳膊上用刀割开皮肉刮骨，发出沙沙的声音，关羽的手下们都大惊失色，而关羽却饮酒吃肉下棋，谈笑如常，完全没有丝毫痛苦的神色。华佗为关羽刮去骨上之毒，敷上伤药，进行缝合。手术之后，关羽的右臂很快就能伸展自如了。

这个故事流传甚广，那么乌头究竟是什么呢？故事里的乌头就是川乌。其实，有毒的乌头也是一味中药，因为它的主根呈圆锥状，看起来就像乌鸦的头一样，因此得名乌头。乌头毒性很强，相传古人把它制成箭毒，中箭者射中即倒。

现代研究证明，乌头中含有有毒的乌头碱，然而只要炮制得法和用量适宜，就能发挥良好的治疗作用，有祛风散寒的功效，因此是医家常用药材。

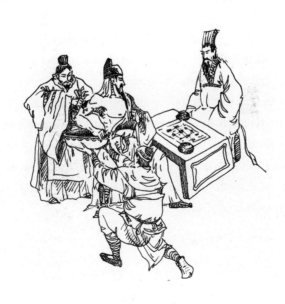

Story

You must have heard the story in *Romance of the Three Kingdoms* that Hua Tuo treated Guan Yu by scraping the poison off the bone. The story is like this: when Guan Yu was leading his army to conquer Fancheng, he was shot by a poisonous arrow in his right arm. After Hua Tuo's examination, he found that Guan Yu was injured by the toxin from Wutou and he could only be cured by scraping the toxin from his bone. The operation was performed with the consent of Guan Yu. Hua Tuo cut the skin and flesh on Guan Yu's right arm and scraped the bone with a knife, making a rustling sound. The soldiers on the scene were all in a panic. However, Guan Yu was drinking wine and eating meat while playing chess, talking and laughing as usual, showing no sign of pain. Meanwhile, Hua Tuo scraped off the poison on the bone, applied wound medicine and sewed it up. After the operation, Guan Yu's right arm soon recovered.

This story is very popular, but what exactly is Wutou? Wutou in the story is Chuanwu. Actually, poisonous Wutou is also a Chinese herbal medicine. Because its main root is conical and looks like the head of a crow, it is named Wutou (which literally means the head of a crow). Wutou is highly toxic. Ancient people made it into arrow poison, and people or animals that got shot would fall down immediately.

Modern research has proved that Wutou contains the aconitine which is toxic. However, with the right processing method and appropriate dosage, it can play a good therapeutic role and have the effect of dispelling wind and cold, so it is a medicinal material commonly used by doctors.

丹参

Danshen / Danshen Root / Radix Salviae Miltiorrhizae

知识模块

来源：唇形科（Labiatae）植物丹参 *Salviae miltiorrhiza* Bge. 的干燥根和根茎。

产地：主产于安徽、江苏、山东、河北、陕西和四川等地。

本草始载：始载于东汉《神农本草经》。

功效：活血祛瘀，凉血消痈，除烦安神。

主治：治疗各种瘀血证，心烦不眠，疮痈肿毒。对心血管疾病疗效较好。

Basic knowledge

Origin: The dry root and rhizome of *Salviae miltiorrhiza* Bge. belonging to the family Labiatae.

Location: Danshen is mainly produced in Anhui, Jiangsu, Shandong, Hebei, Shannxi, and Sichuan provinces, etc.

First recorded in: *Shennong's Classic of Materia Medica* of the Eastern Han Dynasty.

Efficacy: Activating blood circulation to dispel stasis, cooling blood for eliminating carbuncles, relieving restlessness and inducing tranquilization.

Indications: Blood stasis, restlessness and insomnia, sores and abscesses, carbuncles and swellings. It has good effects on cardiovascular diseases.

拓展模块

在生活中，丹参也可作茶饮，例如山楂丹参茶，具有活血化瘀之功效，对于心血管的保护作用非常的不错，有利于降血压、降血脂，还可以开胃健脾、健胃消食。女性月经不调或者痛经，也可以适当饮用此茶，有利于缓解症状。

Related information

In life, Danshen can also be used in tea, such as Hawthorn-Danshen tea, which has the effect of activating blood circulation and removing blood stasis. With a very good protective effect on cardiovascular system, it is conducive to lowering blood pressure and blood lipid. Besides,

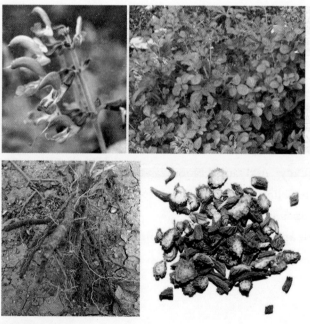

丹参的根真的很红

it can also promote appetite and digestion. Women with irregular menstruation or dysmenorrhea can also drink this tea appropriately, which will help alleviate their symptoms.

故事模块

相传很久以前，东海岸边一个渔村里住着一个名叫阿明的青年。阿明从小丧父，与母亲相依为命。因自幼在风浪中长大，练就了一身好水性，人称"小蛟龙"。

有一年，阿明的母亲患了妇科病，经常崩漏下血，请了很多大夫，都未治愈，阿明一筹莫展。正当此时，有人告诉他东海中有个无名岛，岛上长着一种开紫花、根呈红色的草药，以这种草药的根煎汤内服，就能治愈他母亲的病。阿明听后喜出望外，决定去无名岛采药。可是村里的人听说后，都劝阿明千万不要冒险，因为去无名岛的海路不仅布满暗礁，而且水流湍急，欲上岛者十有九死，犹如闯"鬼门关"一般。但是病不宜迟，阿明救母心切，毅然决定出海上岛采药。

第二天，阿明就驾船出海了。他凭着高超的水性，绕过了一个个暗礁，冲过了一个个激流险滩，终于顺利登上了无名岛。上岸后，他四处寻找那种草药，很快挖了一大捆。返回家后，阿明每日按时侍奉母亲服药，母亲的病很快就痊愈了。

村里人对阿明非常敬佩，都说这种草药凝结了阿明的一片丹心，便给这种长着红色根的草药取名"丹心"。后来在流传过程中，取其谐音就变成"丹参"了。虽然这只是一个传说，但也体现出中华民族崇尚孝道的优良传统。

Story

It is said that a long time ago, a young man named A-Ming lived in a fishing village on the coast of the East Sea. A-Ming lost his father in childhood, so he lived with his mother and they depended on each other. As he grew up near the sea, he developed excellent skills in swimming and sailing, so he was well-known as "Little Dragon".

One year, A-Ming's mother suffered from a gynecological disease named metrorrhagia. A-Ming took his mother to visit many doctors, but none of them cured her disease. A-Ming was really worried and helpless. At this time, some people told him that there was an unnamed island in the East Sea. On this island, there was a kind of herb with purple flowers and red roots. The root of this herb can be used to cure his mother's disease. Hearing that, A-Ming immediately decided to go to the island to collect the root of this special herb. A large number of villagers all advised A-Ming not to take the risk, because the route to the unknown island was full of dangers, including fatal reefs and fast-flowing currents. Many people who wanted to get to the island lost their lives halfway, so the island got the nickname "Gate of Hell". But A-Ming was determined and would not listen to their warning.

The next day, A-Ming sailed out to sea. With the superb sailing skills, he bypassed many fatal reefs and sailed through the dangerous currents and finally landed on the island. After landing, he looked around for the special herb, and soon he collected a large bunch of them. After returning home, A-Ming prepared the medicine on time every day, and his mother recovered quickly after taking the medicine.

The people in the village admire A-Ming very much. They all said that this herb was a symbol of his obedient heart, so they named it "Dan Xin" (which literally means "red heart", a symbol of loyalty in Chinese). Later, in the process of circulation, the name was changed into "Danshen". Though this is just a folktale, it shows people in China attach great importance to filial piety, which is one of the fine traditions of Chinese nation.

甘草

Gancao / Liquorice Root / Radix Glycyrrhizae

知识模块

来源：豆科（Leguminosae）植物甘草 *Glycyrrhizae uralensis* Fisch.、胀果甘草 *G. inflata* Bat. 或光果甘草 *G. glabra* L. 的干燥根及根茎。

产地：主产于我国东北、西北及华北地区。

本草始载：始载于东汉《神农本草经》。

功效：能补中益气，清热解毒，祛痰止咳，缓急止痛，调和药性。

主治：治疗脾胃虚弱证，咳嗽气喘，心悸气短，痈肿疮毒，缓解药物毒性和烈性。

Basic knowledge

Origin: The dry root and rhizome of *Glycyrrhizae uralensis* Fisch., *G. inflata* Bat. or *G. glabra* L. belonging to the family Leguminosae.

Location: Gancao is mainly produced in Northeast China, Northwest China and North China.

First recorded in: *Shennong's Classic of Materia Medica* of the Eastern Han Dynasty.

Efficacy: Invigorating spleen-stomach and replenishing qi, clearing heat and toxicity, eliminating phlegm and relieving cough, relieving spasm pain, harmonizing medicinal properties.

Indications: Spleen and stomach deficiency syndrome, cough and asthma, palpitations, shortness of breath, sore and abscess. It can also relieve toxic property or violent property of some herbs.

植物甘草耐旱、耐盐碱，根系发达，是西北重要的固沙植物，对保护当地生态环境发挥积极作用。甘草作为一味常用中药，有着"十方九草"的美誉，大量用于临床配方。此外，甘草被收载于《既是食品又是药品的物品名单》，可以作为普通食品的原料或添加剂，例如酸甜爽口的甘草杏。生活中可以用甘草搭配不同的食材和药材煮汤，起到不错的保健作用，比如绿豆甘草汤、甘草蜜枣汤、大麦甘草茶等。再者，甘草中的黄酮类成分还有美白的作用，被广泛添加到化妆品中。

Related information

Gancao herb is drought-tolerant and salt-tolerant with well-developed roots, so it is an important sand-fixing plant in the northwest of China and plays a positive role in protecting the local ecological environment. Gancao, as a commonly used medicine, enjoys a reputation of "shi fang jiu cao" (which means it is applied in nine out of ten prescriptions) because it is used in a large amount of clinic prescriptions. In addition, Gancao is included in List of Items That Are Both Food and Medicine and can be used as an ingredient or additive in some foods, such as licorice apricot which is quite refreshing with the sour and sweet

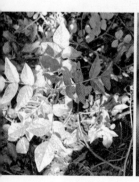
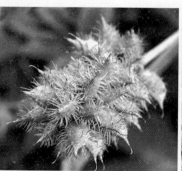
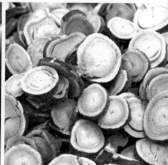

taste. In daily life, people can also cook soup or make tea with Gancao and different ingredients or medicines for health care, such as mung bean-Gancao soup, Gancao-candied date soup, barley-Gancao tea, and so on. Finally, the flavonoids in Gancao also have a whitening effect and are widely applied in cosmetics.

故事模块

甘草是一味人们非常熟悉的中药，治疗咳嗽常用的西药"复方甘草片"就是以甘草为主要成分。甘草素有"国老"之称，这个说法据说是由陶弘景最先提出来的。

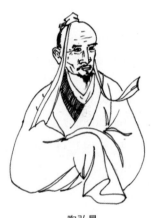

陶弘景

陶弘景是我国南朝齐、梁时期著名医药学家。梁武帝年间，陶弘景隐居在句曲山（即现在江苏省的茅山）上，潜心修道，并婉拒了梁武帝的多次入朝为官的邀请，但是朝廷中每遇大事皇帝便会派人向他咨询，所以当时人们称陶弘景为"山中宰相"。

一天，梁武帝又派侍从来到句曲山，请陶弘景火速面君。原来，梁武帝连日来不思饮食，上吐下泻，朝中的御医们会诊无效，梁武帝便想到了陶弘景，他深知陶弘景知识广博，不仅上知天文下知地理，尤其是在医学方面造诣更为精深。

陶弘景给梁武帝诊脉后，便开了处方，里面有一味药是"国老"，御医们看了后都不知"国老"是什么药。陶弘景笑着说："国老者，甘草之美称也。甘草调和众药，使之不争，堪称国老矣。"众御医听了都点头称赞。果然梁武帝经过陶弘景的诊治，身体日渐康复。

Story

Gancao is a kind of Chinese herbal medicine which is very familiar to people. For example, it is a main ingredient of "Fufang Gancao Pian" (Compound Liquorice Tablets), a Western medicine commonly used to treat cough. Gancao is known as "Guo Lao" (which means an important minister of the country). This term is said to have been first put forward by Tao Hongjing.

Tao Hongjing was a famous medical scientist in the Qi and Liang periods of the Northern and Southern Dynasties (420−589). During the reign of Emperor Wu, Tao Hongjing lived in seclusion on Juqu Mountain (now Maoshan Mountain of Jiangsu Province), devoting himself to Taoism. He refused politely many times the invitation of Emperor Wu to work in the imperial court. However, the emperor would send people to consult him whenever major events took place in the country, so people at that time called Tao Hongjing "Chancellor in Mountains".

One day, the emperor sent his attendants to invite Tao Hongjing to meet him in the palace quickly. It turned out that the emperor was sick with a poor appetite, and suffered from serious vomiting and diarrhea. After the failure of the royal doctors, the emperor sent for Tao Hongjing because he knew that Tao Hongjing was not only knowledgeable, but also skilled in medicine.

Tao Hongjing gave the emperor a prescription after checking his pulse. There was a medicine called "Guo Lao" in the prescription. The royal doctors were all puzzled what it was. Tao Hongjing said with a smile, "Guo Lao here is Gancao. Since Gancao can harmonize other medicines, that's why it's called Guo Lao." After hearing this, all the royal doctors nodded their heads in praise. Sure enough, the emperor recovered gradually after Tao Hongjing's treatment.

白芍

Baishao / Debark Peony Root / Radix Paeoniae Alba

知识模块

来源：芍药科（Paeoniaceae）植物芍药 *Paeonia lactiflora* Pall. 的干燥根。

产地：主产于华东地区及四川等地。其原植物为栽培品种。

本草始载：始载于东汉《神农本草经》。

功效：养血调经，平肝止痛。

主治：治疗血虚，月经不调，自汗，盗汗等症，同时具有一定的保肝作用。

Basic knowledge

Origin: The dry root of *Paeonia lactiflora* Pall. belonging to the family Paeoniaceae.

Location: Baishao is mainly produced in East China and Sichuan Province, etc. The plant is a cultivar.

First recorded in: *Shennong's Classic of Materia Medica* of the Eastern Han Dynasty.

Efficacy: Tonifying blood, regulating menstruation, suppressing hyperactive liver for alleviating pain.

Indications: Blood deficiency, irregular menstruation, spontaneous sweating, night sweats and other symptoms. It can also protect the liver.

拓展模块

芍药一直是中国古代著名的花卉。传说芍药原本并不是尘世间的花，某年人间瘟疫泛滥，善良的花神为拯救世人而盗取了王母的仙丹撒下人

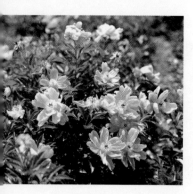
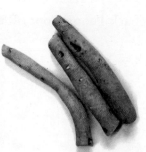
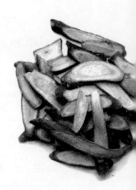

间。结果有一些仙丹就变成了草本的芍药，所以芍药的名字中有个"药"字。芍药观赏价值极高，是我国传统名贵花卉，素有"花相"之称，排名仅次于"花王"牡丹。

白芍被收载于《可用于保健食品的物品名单》。它可以用来泡水喝，也可以做药膳，比如白芍炖猪肘、白芍炖乳鸽等。再比如"四物汤"是一道传统药膳，以当归、川芎、白芍、熟地黄四味药材熬制而成，是中医补血、养血的经典药膳。但白芍性寒，因此虚寒性腹痛泄泻者不宜食用。

Related information

Shaoyao (paeonia lactiflora) has always been a famous flower in ancient China. Legend has it that it was not a flower from the human's world. One year, a plague struck the world, and in order to save the people, the kind-hearted Goddess of Flowers stole some magic drugs from the Heavenly Queen Mother, and scattered them to the human's world. As a result, some of the magic drugs turned into Shaoyao, that's how Shaoyao got its name ("yao" means "medicine" in Chinese). Besides medicinal value, Shaoyao also has a very high ornamental value, and it is a traditional and precious flower of our country. It is known as the "chancellor of flowers", right after peony, the "king of flowers".

Baishao is included in List of Items That Can Be Used as Health Food. It can be soaked in water for people to drink, or can be made in herbal cuisine, such as stewed pork knuckle or pigeon with Baishao. Another example is "Siwu Tang", which is a traditional medicinal diet. It is made with Danggui (Chinese angelica), Chuanxiong (Szechuan lovage rhizome), Baishao and Shudihuang (prepared rehmannia root) as the main ingredients. It is the classic Chinese medicinal diet for tonifying and nourishing blood. But Baishao is cold in nature, so people with abdominal pain or diarrhea due to deficiency-cold had better not take it.

故事模块

相传神医华佗喜欢在院中栽种各种草药，以便研究他们的药性，更好地为病人治疗疾病。有一次，有人送给他一棵芍药，华佗把它种在了屋前。到了春天，华佗尝了尝这棵芍药的叶、茎、花之后，觉得没有什么特殊之处，就没再去管它。

一天深夜，华佗正在灯下看书，突然听到门外有女子的啼哭声。华佗非常纳闷，于是推门走出去，却不见人影，只见那棵芍药兀自挺立。华佗心中一动：难道它就是刚才啼哭的女子？他看了看芍药花，摇了摇头，自言自语地说："你全身上下并无奇特之处，怎能入药呢？"转身又回屋看书去了。

谁知刚刚坐下，又听见那女子的啼哭声，出去看时，还是那棵芍药。华佗觉得奇怪，就将刚才发生的事给妻子描述了一遍。妻子对他说："这里的一草一木，到你手里都成了救人的良药，唯独这株芍药被冷落在一旁，它自然感到委屈了。"

华佗听罢笑道："我尝尽了百草，药性无不辨得一清二楚，没有错过分毫。对这芍药，我也多次尝过了它的叶、茎、花，确实不能入药，怎么说是委屈了它呢？"

　　事隔几日，华夫人血崩腹痛，用药无效。她瞒着丈夫，挖起芍药根煎水喝了。不过半日，腹痛渐止。她把此事告诉了丈夫，华佗才知道他确实委屈了芍药。

　　后来，华佗对芍药做了细致的试验，发现它不但可以<u>止血</u>、<u>活血</u>，而且有镇痛、滋补、调经的效果。这虽然是个传说，但也说明我国古人很早就认识到芍药的药用价值了。

Story

　　According to legend, Hua Tuo, an ancient master of TCM, liked to plant herbs in his yard and studied their medicinal properties in order to better treat various diseases. Once, someone gave him a plant named Shaoyao, and Hua Tuo planted it in front of the house. In the spring, after Hua Tuo tasted the leaves, stems and flowers of this herb, he felt that there was nothing special about it, so from then on he seldom paid attention to it.

　　One night, when Hua Tuo was reading books, he suddenly heard a woman crying outside the door. He opened the door, but did not see anyone in the yard. Only the Shaoyao was standing upright there. Hua Tuo wondered: is it possible that the Shaoyao made the crying sound? He looked closely at the flower again and shook his head; then he spoke to it, "I didn't find any medical value in you. How can I apply you in my prescriptions?" Then he entered the house and began to read again.

　　But just as he sat down, the crying started again. He came out to the yard for the second time, but still saw nothing else but the Shaoyao standing alone in the yard. Hua Tuo felt strange, and told his wife about this. "In your hands," his wife said, "most of the grasses and woods you planted here turned into medicines which can heal and save people. Only this Shaoyao is left out, so it feels being wronged."

Hearing this, Hua Tuo smiled and said, "I have tasted plenty of herbs, and can tell their medicinal properties very clearly. As for this Shaoyao, I have tasted its leaves, stems and flowers for many times, and it proves that it really cannot be used as a medicine. How can you say that it has been wronged? "

A few days later, Mrs. Hua suffered from metrorrhagia with abdominal pain, and the prescriptions proved to be useless. Without telling her husband, she dug out the roots of Shaoyao, decocted it and drank the soup. Only after half a day, her abdominal pain gradually faded away. She told her husband about this, and Hua Tuo knew that he had indeed wronged the Shaoyao.

Later, Hua Tuo made a detailed test on the Shaoyao, and found that it not only could stop bleeding and promote blood, but also had the effects of pain-killing, nourishing and menstruation adjusting. Though this is just a legend, it shows that the people in ancient time have already known the medical values of Shaoyao.

半夏

Banxia / Pinellia Tuber / Rhizoma Pinelliae

来源： 天南星科（Araceae）植物半夏 *Pinellia ternata* (Thunb.) Breit. 的干燥块茎。

产地： 主产于四川、湖北、河南、贵州和安徽等地。

本草始载： 始载于东汉《神农本草经》。

功效： 燥湿化痰，降逆止呕。

主治： 治疗痰湿呕吐、反胃、咳嗽痰多，胸膈胀满。

Basic knowledge

Origin: The dry tuber of *Pinellia ternata* (Thunb.) Breit. belonging to the family Araceae.

Location: Banxia is mainly produced in Sichuan, Hubei, Henan, Guizhou, and Anhui provinces, etc.

First recorded in: *Shennong's Classic of Materia Medica* of the Eastern Han Dynasty.

Efficacy: Drying dampness and resolving phlegm, descending adverse rise of qi and stopping vomiting.

Indications: Vomiting due to phlegm-damp, nausea, cough, phlegm, epigastric stuffiness.

拓展模块

半夏在中药宝库占有一席之地，能够化痰止咳，对于恶心呕吐、胸脘痞闷、疮疡肿痛等症有较好的疗效。但是要注意，生半夏有毒，被载入《保健食品禁用物品名单》。因此生半夏需要炮制后使用。根据不同炮制方法有姜半夏、法半夏、清半夏等规格。

Related information

Banxia occupies a place in the treasure house of Chinese herbal medicines. It can dissipate phlegm and relieve cough. It has a good effect on nausea and vomiting, chest tightness, sores and abscesses. But it is worth noting that raw Banxia is poisonous and is included in List of Items That Are Prohibited in Health Food. Therefore, it needs to be processed before being used. According to different processing methods, there are Jiang Banxia, Fa Banxia and Qing Banxia.

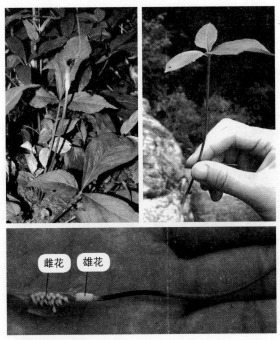

半夏的花是雌雄同株

　　宋朝时期，有位名叫杨立之的官员在南方做官，后来回到老家时得了喉痈（类似于西医中的急性扁桃体炎），白天疼得吃不下饭，晚上痛得睡不着觉，异常痛苦。他的两个儿子请了许多医生，吃了许多中药都没见效。

　　恰好这时一位知名太医杨吉老来这里办事，杨立之的两个儿子听说后，赶紧把他请了过来。太医仔细诊察了杨立之很久后才对他的两个儿子说："你父亲必须先吃一斤生姜片，才可以用药，否则便无法可治！"说完就告辞去办事了。

　　两个儿子感到很为难，因为父亲的喉咙已经溃烂，疼痛不止，怎么还能吃生姜这种辛辣的东西呢？但因为没有别的办法，只好按照太医说的试一试。杨立之忍着疼痛吃了很多生姜片。没过多久，果然喉咙不像先前那么疼了。到了第二天，他已经可以正常地吃饭喝汤了。

　　杨立之马上亲自去拜谢太医，感谢他的救命之恩，并询问是什么原因引起了自己的这种急症。太医

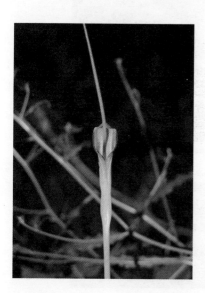

说："昨天你曾跟我说，你在南方做官时很爱吃鹧鸪肉，而鹧鸪爱吃野生的半夏。生半夏具有一定的毒性，你吃鹧鸪吃得多了，就容易引起生半夏中毒，因此会感觉喉咙剧痛。而生姜恰好能解生半夏的毒性，所以我仅用生姜就把你的病根儿除了。"

　　由此可知，生半夏有一定毒性，一定要经过炮制后才能使用，而且生半夏不适合长期服用。不管是医生还是病人都要切记，切记！

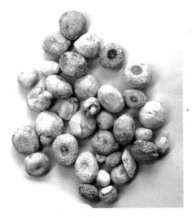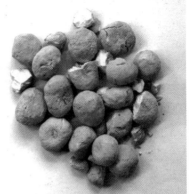

Story

During the Song Dynasty, a government official named Yang Lizhi had worked in the South for quite a long time. When he returned to his hometown, he suffered from a severe throat abscess (similar to acute tonsillitis in Western medicine). Unable to eat during the day and sleep well at night, he was extremely painful. His two sons have invited many doctors, but none of them can cure the disease.

By coincidence, a well-known royal doctor named Yang Jilao came to his hometown. Hearing about that, the two sons of Yang Lizhi invited the doctor to treat their father. The doctor carefully examined Yang Lizhi for a long time and said to his two sons, "Your father must eat a pound of ginger slices before I can use other medicine, otherwise the disease will not be cured." Then the doctor went away to do his own business.

The two sons hesitated because their father's throat was already festering and the pain was severe. How could he eat the spicy things like ginger? But there was no other choice, and they had to try the doctor's instruction. Bearing the severe pain, Yang Lizhi took a large amount of ginger. It didn't take long for him to feel less painful. By the next day, he could eat food and drink soup as normal.

He immediately went to thank the doctor. After expressing his gratitude, he asked the doctor the cause of his disease. The doctor said, "You told me yesterday that you loved to eat francolin meat when you worked in the South. And the francolins love to eat the wild Banxia which is toxic. Their meat also has certain toxicity, so the more you eat francolin meat, the more likely you will get poisoned. That is the major cause of your severe pain in the throat. Ginger is able to dissolve the toxicity of Banxia; that is why I asked you to eat plenty of ginger."

It can be seen that the unprocessed Banxia has certain toxicity, so it must be processed before being used, and it is not suitable for long-term use. Whether you are a doctor or a patient, always bear this in mind.

百合
Baihe / Lily Bulb / Bulbus Lilii

来源： 百合科（Liliaceae）植物百合 *Lilium brownii* F. E. Brown var. *viridulum* Baker、卷丹 *L. lancifolium* Thunb. 或细叶百合 *L. pumilum* DC. 的肉质鳞茎。

产地： 在全国各地均有生产，但是主要产自浙江、湖南等地。

本草始载： 始载于东汉《神农本草经》。

功效： 养阴润肺，止咳化痰，清心安神。

主治： 治疗肺阴虚证以及心神不宁的失眠。

Basic knowledge

Origin: The fleshy bud scale of *Lilium brownii* F. E. Brown var. *viridulum* Baker, *L. lancifolium* Thunb., or *L. pumilum* DC. belonging to the family Liliaceae.

Location: Baihe is cultivated in most parts of China, but the biggest output comes from Zhejiang and Hunan provinces.

First recorded in: *Shennong's Classic of Materia Medica* of the Eastern Han Dynasty.

Efficacy: Nourishing yin and moistening lung, relieving cough and dissipating phlegm, calming heart and inducing tranquilization.

Indications: Lung yin deficiency syndromes, insomnia caused by restlessness.

拓展模块

百合花是生活中常见的一种花卉，受到很多人的喜爱。百合除了作为观赏植物之外，它的肉质鳞茎还可以作为一种中药材来使用，能够起到清热解毒、润肺滋阴、止咳化痰、清心安神、止血止痛等作用。此外，百合也是生活中常用的食材，被载于《既是食品又是药品的物品名单》，可用来煮粥、做菜、炖汤，比如西芹炒百合，百合莲子粥等都是人们喜欢的美食。目前市场上的食用百合主要是兰州百合，因为昼夜温差大，所以积累了大量糖分，是百合中唯一的甜百合。但风寒咳嗽、脾虚便溏者不宜食用百合。

Related information

Lily is a common flower in life, which is loved by many people. In addition to being an ornamental plant, its fleshy bud scale can also be used as a Chinese herbal medicine with the Chinese name Baihe, which can clear heat and toxicity, moisten lung and nourish yin, relieve cough and phlegm, clear heart and calm mind, stop bleeding and stop pain. In addition, Baihe is also commonly used in daily life, and is included in List of Items That Are both Food and Medicne. For example, it can

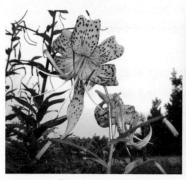

卷丹

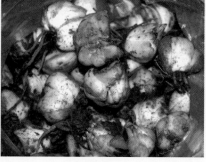

百合的鳞茎

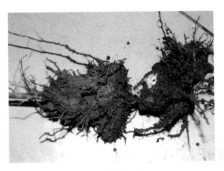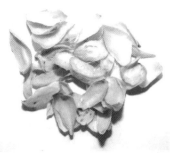

刚挖出来的鳞茎

be cooked in porridge, stir fried, or stewed in soup, such as "Stir-Fried Celery and Lily Bulbs", and "lily bulbs and lotus seed porridge" which are very popular. At present, the main edible Baihe on the market is Lanzhou Baihe. The temperature difference between day and night in Lanzhou is large, so it accumulates a large amount of sugar, which makes it the only sweet Baihe. However, the people with wind-cold, cough, spleen deficiency and loose stool had better not take it.

故事模块

　　相传，曾经有一伙海盗打劫一个渔村，除了把渔民家里的钱财洗劫一空外，还把百余名妇女儿童劫持走，带到大海中的一个孤岛上。过了几天，海盗又去出海打劫，海上突然刮起了台风，海盗们都葬身海底。孤岛上没有船只，妇女和儿童都没法逃跑。半个月后，粮食便被他们吃完了，他们只得挖野菜采野果充饥。有一次，他们挖来一种草根，圆圆的，像大蒜一样，根块肉厚肥实，便把它们洗干净放到锅里煮熟，一尝还有点香甜味。此后，他们就一直采挖这种草根来充饥。

　　一天，有只船来到孤岛上。船上的采药人听说了他们的经历，看到这些儿童都吃得胖乎乎的，妇女们也满脸丰盈红润，便断定这是一种有营养的药草。经过验证，这种草根不仅能够润肺止咳，还可以清心安神。因考虑到这种草根是百余名妇女儿童合力采挖品尝后才发现的，所以，采药人就给它起了个名字叫"百合"。

当然这只是一个传说故事。其实百合的食用和药用部位可不是它的根，而是它的地下鳞茎，看着像大蒜头，剥开后是一层层的鳞片，经过烘干后制成百合干片，有食用和药用两种功效。并不是所的百合都可以食用，像平时所见的香水百合等，常用于观赏或插花；可食用的品种有兰州百合、卷丹百合等。

Story

According to legend, there was a group of pirates who robbed a fishing village. In addition to looting the fishermen's money, they also hijacked more than a hundred women and children, and took them to an isolated island in the sea. After a few days, the pirates went out to rob by boat, but all the pirates were drowned in the sea because of typhoon. There were no boats on the island, so the women and children couldn't escape. After half a month, they ran out of food. Then they had to dig wild herbs and picked wild fruits to appease hunger. Once, they dug out a kind of round grassroots, which looked like thick and fat garlic. They washed them clean and boiled them as food. The grassroots tasted very sweet, and most people on the island liked eating them. Since then, they began to feed on this plant.

One day, a boat arrived on the island. The medicinal herb collectors on the ship heard about their experiences. They saw that these children were chubby, and the women were also full of energy and enjoyed rosy cheeks, and they concluded that it was a nutritious herbal medicine. Later, it was proven that this kind of grass root can not only moisten the lungs and relieve cough, but also clear the heart and calm the nerves.

Because the grass roots were discovered and dug out by the joint efforts of more than a hundred women and children, it got the name "Bai He" (which literally means "joint efforts of one hundred people").

Of course, it's just a legend story. Actually, the edible and medicinal part of lily is not its root, but its underground bulb. It looks like a head of garlic. After peeling, you can see layers of scales. After drying, they are made into dried lily bulb slices which are both food and medicine. Not all lily species are edible. Many lily varieties are commonly used for ornament or flower arranging such as Lilium Casa Blanca. Edible varieties include Lanzhou lily (*Lilium davidii* var. unicolor) and tiger lily (*Lilium lancifolium* Thunb.), etc.

当归
Danggui / Chinese Angelica / Radix Angelicae Sinensis

来源： 伞形科（Umbelliferae）植物当归 *Angelica sinensis* (Oliv.) Diels 的干燥根。

产地： 产于甘肃岷县等地。

本草始载： 始载于东汉《神农本草经》。

功效： 能补血活血，调经止痛，润肠通便。

主治： 治疗血虚证，妇科月经不调，经闭痛经，肠燥便秘。

Basic knowledge

Origin: The dry root of *Angelica sinensis* (Oliv.) belonging to the family Umbelliferae.

Location: Danggui is mainly produced in Minxian County of Gansu Province, etc.

First recorded in: *Shennong's Classic of Materia Medica* of the Eastern Han Dynasty.

Efficacy: Tonifying blood and promoting blood circulation, regulating menstruation and relieving pain, laxative.

Indications: Syndrome of blood deficiency, irregular menstruation, amenorrhea, dysmenorrhea, constipation due to intestinal dryness.

拓展模块

当归常用于妇女血虚，月经不调，虚寒腹痛等。被誉为"补血第一药"。除药用外，它还作为保健品使用，收录于《可用于保健食品的物品名单》。我国民间常用当归配合其他食材煲汤，能起到很好的保健养生作用，比如早在东汉时期，张仲景就在《金匮要略》中记载了血虚内寒者可用当归生姜羊肉汤进行调理，做法也很简单，当归三两，生姜三两，羊肉一斤，加水炖汤，在寒冷的冬季可用来食疗强身，尤其可以用来产后及失血后调理身体。

Related information

Danggui is often used for women with blood deficiency, irregular menstruation, asthenia, abdominal pain due to cold deficiency, etc. It is known as "the first medicine for tonifying blood". In addition to medicinal uses, it also can be used as a health product and is included in List of Items That Can Be Used as Health Food. As early as the Eastern Han Dynasty, for example, Zhang Zhongjing recorded in the *Synopsis of the Golden Chamber* that people with blood deficiency and internal cold could use Danggui-mutton Soup to help keep healthy. The recipe is very simple: just stew soup with 150 grams of Danggui, 150 grams of ginger, and 1 kilogram of mutton. This soup is very beneficial for people in cold winter, especially for postpartum women or people who have lost much blood.

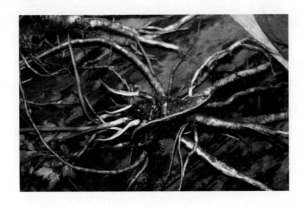

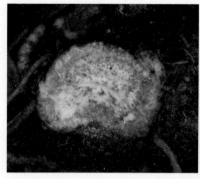
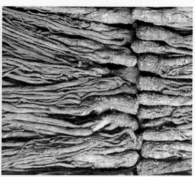

故事模块

说起当归，有很多与它有关的历史故事和民间传说。

三国时期，司马昭派遣大将进攻蜀国，蜀国后主刘禅昏庸无能开门投降，蜀国大将姜维在无可奈何之下只得假意投降，打算积蓄力量，以便日后复兴蜀国。后来，司马昭派人抓去了姜维的母亲。姜维的母亲得知儿子投降后气愤难耐，写了一封信斥责姜维不忠不孝不义。姜维看到母亲的信后心中十分忐忑不安，如果不对母亲说出实情，母亲会一直错怪他，如果对母亲说出实话，又担心泄露天机坏了大事。正当他左右为难之际，他突然想到一个绝妙的方法。他拿了两包中药，一包是远志，另一包是当归，托人送给母亲。姜维的母亲看后，马上心领神会，完全理解了儿子的用意。于是，为了让姜维毫无牵挂，自己便撞墙而死。

关于当归名字的由来，还相传与一个"当归不归，娇妻改嫁"的故事有关。相传，有个新婚青年上山采药，对妻子说三年回来。媳妇因思念丈夫而忧郁悲伤，得了气血亏损的妇科病。三年期满却仍不见丈夫归来，她以为丈夫已经身亡便只好改嫁。谁知后来丈夫却又回来了，他看到妻子已经改嫁他人，非常懊悔自己没有按时归来，遂把采集的草药根拿去给媳妇治病，没想竟然治好了她的妇科病。此后这种药就被称为"当归"。

Story

When it comes to Danggui, there are many historical stories and folklores about it.

During the Three Kingdoms Period（220-280）, Sima Zhao from Wei State sent army to attack Shu State. Liu Chan, the cowardly King of Shu State, was so afraid that he surrendered. Jiang Wei, the Major General of Shu State, had no choice but to pretend to surrender, hoping to keep his army in order to revive Shu State in the future. Later Sima Zhao sent people to capture Jiang Wei's mother as a threat to Jiang Wei. Jiang Wei's mother was very angry when she learned that her son had surrendered, so she wrote a letter to denounce Jiang Wei for betraying his state. Jiang Wei felt uneasy when reading his mother's letter. He was in a dilemma: if he didn't tell his mother the truth, he would still be misunderstood, but if he told the truth, he was afraid that his secret would be leaked to the enemy. Suddenly he got a good idea. He took two packages of Chinese herbal medicine, one was Yuanzhi (which literally means "ambition") and the other was Danggui

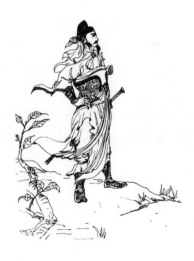

(which literally means "should return"), and sent them to his mother. When Jiang Wei's mother saw it, she immediately understood his son's intentions. Then she killed herself by hitting her head on the wall so that she wouldn't be a burden to her son.

As for the origin of the name of Danggui, it is said to be related to the folklore that "the beautiful wife will remarry if the husband doesn't return". Legend has it that a newly married young man went up to the mountains to collect medicinal herbs. He told his wife that he would return three years later. His wife missed him so much that she got some gynecological diseases due to deficiency of qi and blood. Three years later her husband didn't come back as he had promised, so she thought her husband was already dead and she had no choice but to remarry. However, the husband came back unexpectedly. Seeing that his wife had remarried, he was very sorry that he did not come back on time. He gave the herbal roots that he had collected to his ex-wife. And amazingly she recovered soon after taking the medicine. Then this herb was called "Danggui" (which literally means "should return" in Chinese).

防风
Fangfeng / Divaricate Saposhnikovia Root /
Radix Saposhnikoviae

知识模块

来源：伞形科（Umbelliferae）植物防风 *Saposhnikovia divaricata* (Turcz.) Schischk. 的干燥根。

产地：主产于东北、内蒙古、河北和山西等地。

本草始载：始载于东汉《神农本草经》。

功效：发散风寒，祛风胜湿。

主治：用于治疗外感风寒感冒，风寒湿痹，破伤风等。

Basic knowledge

Origin: The dry root of *Saposhnikovia divaricata* (Turcz.) belonging to the family Umbelliferae.

Location: Fangfeng is mainly produced in Northeast China, Inner Mongolia Autonomos Region, Hebei Province, and Shanxi Province, etc.

First recorded in: *Shennong's Classic of Materia Medica* of the Eastern Han Dynasty.

Efficacy: Dispelling wind-cold, expelling wind-damp.

Indications: Exterior wind-cold, wind-damp arthralgia and pain, tetanus, etc.

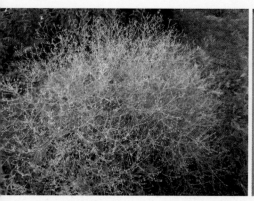
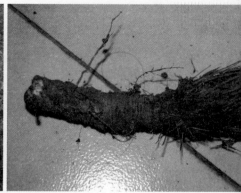

拓展模块

防风性微温而不燥，带有甜味并伴有辛味，在古代也称为"屏风"，意思是能够像屏障一样抵制风寒，常用于治疗风寒感冒，也被用于祛风，祛除湿气。

Related information

Fangfeng, slightly warm in nature but not dry, with sweet and spicy taste, is also called as "Pingfeng" (which literally means screen) in ancient times. It means that it can resist wind and cold like a screen. It is often used to treat wind-cold type common cold, and is also used to dispel wind and dampness.

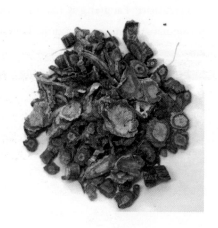

故事模块

防风的故事是流传在浙江省的一则民间神话传说。古防风国位于今天浙江湖州，防风氏是当时的部落领袖，和大禹处于同一个时代，曾跟随大禹治理水患，并立下了汗马功劳。

传说大禹治水成功后，在会稽（今浙江绍兴）召集天下各路诸侯，论功行赏，并且商议以后的治国大计。各州省诸侯纷纷赶到庆贺，庆功大会一连开了三天，却一直不见防风氏的身影，直到庆功会快结束时，防风氏才匆匆赶到。

大禹质问防风氏为何迟到，防风氏说自己在路上遇到了洪水才迟到的。可是大禹在庆功会上一连三天听惯了人们的歌功颂德，他以为防风氏居功自傲，瞧不起自己，于是一怒之下，便下令杀了防风氏。当防风氏的头颅掉落时，伤口却喷出股股白血，散落在山野里，长出一种羽状叶的小草。大禹和诸侯们都很震惊，大禹便派人查问，发现果然是自己冤枉了防风氏。大禹心中十分愧疚，于是便追封防风氏为"防风王"，并为他建立起"防风祠"。

后来，当百姓们受了风寒而感到头晕脑涨、浑身酸痛时，就采来这种小草煎水服下，果然病就好了。乡亲们都说："这是防风神留给我们的神草，就叫它'防风'吧！"

Story

The story of Fangfeng is a folk legend popular in Zhejiang Province. The ancient Fangfeng Kingdom was located in today's Huzhou of Zhejiang province. Fangfeng was the tribal leader at that time. He was in the same era with Dayu (the great leader known as the Tamer of the Flood). He had followed Dayu to control floods and made great contributions.

Legend has it that after Dayu successfully controlled the great flood, all the leaders of different tribes gathered in Kuaiji (now Shaoxing, Zhejiang Province) to celebrate the great achievements of Dayu, and to discuss the grand plans of governing the country in the future. The feast was held for three consecutive days, but Fangfeng didn't show himself at the feast. Until the end of the festival, Fangfeng arrived in a hurry. In a fury, Dayu asked Fangfeng why he was so late. Fangfeng explained that he was late because he was caught in a flood on the road. But Dayu had become complacent due to people's flattery at the feast. He thought Fangfeng was so proud that he looked down upon others. Dayu was extremely angry, and ordered Fangfeng to be beheaded. When Fangfeng's head fell, white blood spurted from his neck and scattered in the mountains, and then turned into many grasses with pinnate leaves. Dayu and all the other people were shocked. He sent his men to make an investigation for the truth, and found that he had misunderstood Fangfeng. With guilt in his heart, Dayu conferred him a posthumous title "Fangfeng King" and asked people to build "Fangfeng Temple" for him.

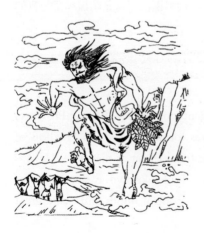

Later, when the local villagers suffered from wind-cold with dizziness and soreness, they picked this kind of grass and decocted water and drink it. They would soon be cured. The villagers all said, "This is the divine grass that Fangfeng has left us. Let's call it Fangfeng!"

何首乌

Heshouwu / Tuber Fleeceflower Root / Radix Polygoni Multiflori

知识模块

来源：蓼科（Polygonaceae）植物何首乌 *Polygonum multiflorum* Thunb. 的干燥块根。

产地：主产于湖北、贵州、四川等地。

本草始载：始载于宋代《开宝本草》。

功效：制用：补益精血。生用：解毒，截疟，润肠通便。

主治：治疗精血亏虚证（制用）；肠燥便秘，皮肤瘙痒等（生用）。

Basic knowledge

Origin: The root tuber of *Polygonum multiflorum* Thunb. belonging to the family Polygonaceae.

Location: Heshouwu is mainly produced in Hubei, Guizhou and Sichuan provinces.

First recorded in: *Kai Bao Ben Cao* (*Materia Medica in Kai-Bao Reign*) of the Song Dynasty.

Efficacy: Processed Heshouwu can tonify blood and supplement essence; unprocessed Heshouwu can relieve toxicity, stop malaria, and moisten dryness for relaxing bowels.

Indications: Processed Heshouwu can treat blood and essence deficiency syndrome; unprocessed Heshouwu can treat constipation due to intestinal dryness, and pruritus.

　　何首乌被古人尊为"九大仙草之一"。何首乌的藤也是中药，叫夜交藤，具有安神和祛风湿的作用。生首乌未经炮制具有泻下作用；而炮制后的何首乌则具有补益作用，这说明中药炮制可以改变药性。同时，虽然何首乌是人们常用的保健药品之一，但有报道称何首乌中的蒽醌类成分会引起肝损害。国家食品药品监督管理总局在 2014 年发文指出，保健食品中生何首乌每日用量不得超过 1.5 g，制何首乌每日用量不得超过 3.0 g，而且肝功能不全者、肝病家族史者不宜使用含何首乌保健食品。

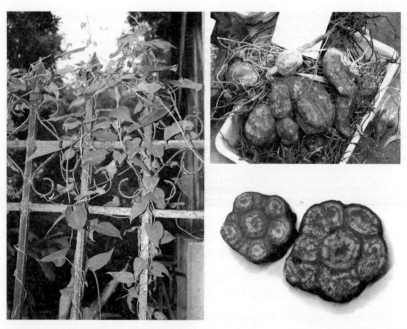

看看何首乌断面上的圆环状结构，药材中叫"云锦花纹"，这是我们鉴别何首乌的最好方法。

Heshouwu was honored by the ancient people as "one of the nine immortal grasses". The vine of Heshouwu is also a Chinese herbal medicine called "Yejiaoteng" with the functions of calming the mind and eliminating rheumatism. The unprocessed Heshouwu has lapactic effect while the processed Heshouwu has tonic effect. This shows that the processing of Chinese herbal medicine can change the properties of medicines. Meanwhile, though Heshouwu is a common health care medicine, it is reported that the anthraquinone compounds in Heshouwu might be harmful to the liver. China Food and Drug Administration issued a document in 2014 which says that the daily dosage of raw Heshouwu in health food should not exceed 1.5g, the daily dosage of processed Heshouwu should not exceed 3.0g, and patients with liver dysfunction or family history of liver disease had better not take the health care food containing Heshouwu.

故事模块

很久以前，有一位名医叫作何朴。他十分精通医术，而且心地善良，为人耿直。有一次，他被恶人陷害，关进了监狱。监狱的看守看他没有什么油水可榨，就不给他吃饭，想活活把他饿死。

何朴饥饿难忍，便在监牢四处走动，想找到一点儿吃的东西。结果他发现监狱的窗外长满了蒿草。由于太饿，何朴想拔些草叶来吃，结果这种蒿草很容易连根拔起。何朴把蒿草拿到牢房里，发现它的根像土豆一样大小，呈土灰色，他把泥土去掉后尝了尝，味道虽然不太好，但却可以用来充饥。就这样，何朴每天拔出几个来吃，一直坚持了好几个月。

后来，有一天夜里，刮起了台风，把本来已经摇摇欲坠的牢房吹倒了。何朴连夜逃跑，在逃跑前还挖了一些蒿草根，以免路上饿肚子。

就这样，何朴翻山越岭，跋山涉水，没过几天就回到了家乡。可是，回到老家后，乡亲们都认不出他了。原来，何朴比坐牢前显得更年轻了，不仅花白的头发和胡子全都变黑了，而且腰板也比原来硬朗，走路也快得像风一样。何朴觉得自己的变化一定和那蒿草根有关。于是，他便把自己带回来的那些蒿草根种植起来，研究其药性，让乡亲们也都可以从中受益。

从那以后，人们就称这种植物为"何首乌"，因为它是由何朴发现的，而且能够让人们的头发变黑。（"首"是指头部，"乌"是黑的意思。）

当然，这只是一个民间故事，生的何首乌可不能像故事里描述的那样服用。如果想用何首乌治疗白发，必须得遵医嘱才行，千万不能擅自服用生何首乌，以免对身体造成损伤。

Story

A long time ago, there was a famous doctor named He Pu. Proficient in medicine, he was also very kind and upright. Once he was framed up by the wicked and was put into prison. The guard of the prison didn't get any money from him, and then decided not to give him any meal.

When He Pu was hungry, he walked around the cell, hoping to find something to eat. As a result, he found that near the window of the cell there was a kind of plant. Because he was too hungry, He Pu wanted to pick some leaves of the plant to eat. He also uprooted the whole plant while picking its leaves. He Pu took it into the cell and found that its roots were as big as potatoes and had gray color. He removed the soil and tasted the roots. Although the taste was not very good, it could still allay his hunger. In this way, in the following months, He Pu pulled out some roots to eat every day.

Then one night, a typhoon broke out, and the crumbling prison cell was blown down. He Pu escaped at night and dug some roots of this plant before he fled, so as to avoid hunger on the road.

He Pu returned to his hometown in a few days. However, most of the villagers could not recognize him, as He Pu looked much younger than before he was put into jail. His white hair and beard turned black. He could stand straighter than before and walk fast like a wind. He Pu believed that the change in his body must be related to the roots he ate in the last few months. So he decided to plant the herb that he brought back and studied its curative effects, so that the fellow villagers could benefit from that.

Since then, people began to call this plant "Heshouwu", because it was discovered by He Pu and could make people's hair black ("shou" means the head, and "wu" means black).

Of course, this is only a folk story. Actually raw Heshouwu cannot be eaten as described in the story. If you want to use Heshouwu to reduce white hair, you had better follow the doctor's advice. Do not take Heshouwu by yourself; otherwise it might damage the body.

贯众

Guanzhong / Rhizoma Dryopteris Crassirhizomae

来源：鳞毛蕨科（Dryopteridaceae）植物粗茎鳞毛蕨 *Dryopteris crassirhizomae* Nakai 的干燥根茎

产地：主产于东北三省。

本草始载：始载于东汉《神农本草经》。

功效：杀虫，清热解毒，止血。

主治：常用于驱除人体寄生虫，如蛔虫、绦虫和钩虫等，并能治疗风热感冒。

Basic knowledge

Origin: The dry rhizome of *Dryopteris crassirhizomae* Nakai belonging to the family Dryopteridaceae.

Location: Guanzhong is mainly produced in the three provinces in Northeast of China (Heilongjiang, Jilin and Liaoning provinces).

First recorded in: *Shennong's Classic of Materia Medica* of the Eastern Han Dynasty.

Efficacy: Expelling parasites, clearing heat and removing toxicity, stopping bleeding.

Indications: Guanzhong is commonly used to expel parasites in the human body, such as roundworm, tapeworm and hookworms; it is also used to treat wind-heat type common cold.

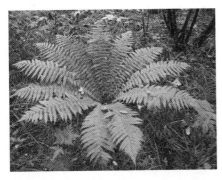 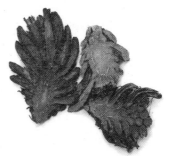

贯众有很多功效，可以清热解毒，对于风热感冒及咽喉肿痛、咳嗽等都有不错的效果；此外，它还能够用来驱除体内的寄生虫。但是，它也有一定的副作用，因此脾胃虚寒者及孕妇等慎用。

Related information

Guanzhong has many functions. For example, it can clear heat and toxicity, and it has a good effect on wind-heat cold, sore throat and cough. In addition, it can also be used to expel parasites in the human body. But it has some side effects, so the patients with deficiency of spleen and stomach and pregnant women had better not use it.

故事模块

从前，有个没有文化的老帮工，一辈子给地主干活。一年夏天，他偶然发现有一种草根能毒死地里的虫子。他想，既然这种草根能杀死土里的虫子，那么它能不能杀死人们肚子里的虫子呢？

有一次，地主家有个儿子生病了，整日不思饮食，日渐消瘦。郎中说孩子体内有几种寄生虫，并给开了一张杀虫的中药处方。可是用过药之后也不见好转，这可把地主给急坏了。老帮工知道了，就偷偷地把他发现的能毒死虫子的草根煎好后，把药汁端给地主的儿子喝。这孩子喝过药之后感觉肚子十分疼痛，几乎昏死过去，这可把老帮工吓坏了。所幸，第二天早饭后，孩子拉出了几十条虫子，肚子也不痛了，也开始想吃东西了。这次老帮工心中有了底：这种草根不但能杀地里的虫子，同样也可以杀肚子里的虫子。于是，他就把这种草根的秘密告诉了大家，使这种药能够造福于普通大众。大家为了向他表示感激，便把这种草根称为"贯众"，意思是"告诉大家"。

Story

Once upon a time, there was an old peasant who worked for the landlord for the most of his life. One summer, he happened to find that the root of a special herb could kill the worms in the field. He thought that since this grass root could kill the worms in the field, was it possible that it could also kill the worms in people's belly?

Once, the son of the landlord fell ill. He had no appetite and gradually got thinner and thinner. The doctor said that there were several parasites in the child's body and prescribed some medicine to expel the parasites. However, the child didn't turn better after taking the medicine, which made the landlord extremely anxious. The old peasant secretly boiled the grass root that he had found, and then gave the soup to the child. After taking the soup, the child felt great pain in his belly and almost fainted, which scared the old peasant. Fortunately, after breakfast the next day, the child excreted dozens of parasites, and his belly did not hurt any more. He began to ask for food. This time the old peasant was sure that this grass root could not only kill the worms in the field, but also kill the parasites in human belly. So he told everyone about the secret of this grass root so that it would benefit the public. In order to express gratitude to him, people named it "Guanzhong", which literally means "to tell the public".

桔梗
Jiegeng / Platycodon Root / Radix Platycodonis

知识模块

来源： 桔梗科（Campanulaceae）植物桔梗 *Platycodon grandiflorus* (Jacq.) A. DC. 的根。

产地： 我国大部分地区均有产地，以东北、华北产量最大。

本草始载： 始载于东汉《神农本草经》。

功效： 宣肺，利咽，祛痰，排脓。

主治： 治疗咳嗽痰多，咽喉肿痛，肺痈吐脓。

Basic knowledge

Origin: The root of *Platycodon grandiflorus* (Jacq.) A. DC. belonging to the family Campanulaceae.

Location: Jiegeng is mainly produced in most areas of China. Northeast China and North China have the biggest output.

First recorded in: *Shennong's Classic of Materia Medica* of the Eastern Han Dynasty.

Efficacy: Ventilating lung qi, relieving sore throat, dispelling phlegm, expelling pus.

Indications: Cough, excessive phlegm, swelling and pain in throat, lung abscess with pyemesis.

你听过著名的朝鲜民歌《道拉基》吗？歌曲中的"道拉基"其实就是指的桔梗花。桔梗一身都是宝，不仅可以制成中药，有宣肺、利咽、祛痰和排脓等功效，它也是一种野菜，被收载于《既是食品又是药品的物品名单》。春夏时节，可以采摘桔梗嫩叶做菜，秋季可以挖出它的根，焯水去除苦味后进行腌制或炒菜。

此外，桔梗开出紫色小花，非常漂亮，也可以作为插花观赏。但是花卉市场上更常见一种叫作"洋桔梗"的花，名字听起来很像是桔梗的"洋姐妹"；但是，事实上，它们可不是同一种植物。桔梗是桔梗科植物，而洋桔梗是龙胆科的植物，常用做盆花和切花，并没有药用价值。

Related information

Have you heard the famous Korean folklore with the name which sounds like *Tao Lachey*? "Tao lachey" in this folklore actually refers to the Jiegeng flower (balloon flower). Jiegeng is very useful because it is not only a medicinal herb with effects of ventilating lung, relieving sore throat, dispelling phlegm, and expelling pus, but also a wild vegetable which is included in List of Items That Are both Food and Medicine. In spring and summer, its tender leaves can be cooked as vegetable, while in autumn its root can be pickled or stir fried after being blanched to get rid of its bitter taste.

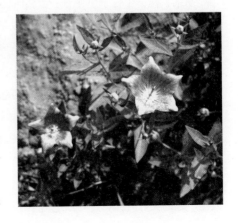

Besides, its purple flowers

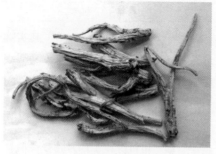
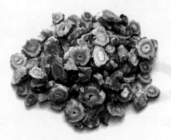

look beautiful and can also be used in flower arranging. However, a flower named "Yang Jiegeng" (which literally means Jiegeng from abroad) is more popular in the flower market. "Yang Jiegeng" sounds like Jiegeng's "sister from abroad", but actually they are quite different. Jiegeng is a plant belonging to the family Campanulaceae which is often used as medicine; while Yang Jiegeng (*Eustoma grandiflorum* (Raf.) Shinners) is a plant belonging to the family Gentianaceae without medicinal effect, and it is often used as pot flower or cut flower.

故事模块

　　从前，在一个村子里住着一位名叫桔梗的少女。她从小就没有父母，无依无靠。有一位和桔梗青梅竹马的少年，对桔梗很是照顾，两人长大后自然就成了一对恋人。但是，小伙子为了生计，不得不乘船去很远的地方捕鱼。他对桔梗说："桔梗啊，一定要等我回来。我一定会回来的！"桔梗与恋人相约在海边，依依不舍地与恋人告别，看着渔船越驶越远，直到消失在海面上，桔梗留下了伤心的泪水。

　　可是，桔梗的恋人却一直没有回来。桔梗经常到海边守望，希望恋人有一天可以回来。就这样过了几十年，桔梗从美丽的少女变成了一位白发老人。这天，她再次来到当初和恋人约定的海边，回忆起以前与恋人在一起的美好时光，她默默地流下了眼泪。然后，她慢慢地闭上眼睛。

突然，她的双脚开始在地上生根，身体则变成了枝丫和鲜花，并且永远朝着大海的方向，等待恋人回来。为了纪念这位少女，人们就把这种花叫作桔梗花，它的花语就是"真诚不变的爱"。

Story

Once upon a time, there was a girl named Jie Geng in a village. Her parents passed away when she was only a child. A boy of her similar age in the village always took good care of her. When they grow up, they became lovers. In order to make a living, one day, the young man had to go to the sea for fishing. He said to his lover, "Jie Geng, wait for me. I will come back." They promised to meet each other at the seaside. Reluctant to part from her lover, Jie Geng bade farewell to him, and shed tears of sorrow seeing that the fishing boat was sailing further and further until it vanished on the sea.

However, for quite a long time, the young man didn't return. Jie Geng often went to the beach, hoping that her lover could come back one day. After several decades, Jie Geng, the once beautiful young girl, became an old lady with white hair. One day, while standing by the seaside, she recalled the good old days with her lover, and then silently shed tears. She slowly closed her eyes. Suddenly, her feet began to take root in the ground, and her body turned into branches and flowers which always faced the sea. To commemorate the girl, people call this flower "Jiegeng" which stands for "true love that never changes".

柴胡

Chaihu / Chinese Thorowax Root / Radix Bupleuri

知识模块

来源：伞形科（Umbelliferae）植物柴胡 *Bupleurum chinensis* DC. 或狭叶柴胡 *B. scorzonerifolium* Willd. 的干燥根。前者习称"北柴胡"，后者习称"南柴胡"。

产地：北柴胡主产于东北、华北；南柴胡主产于湖北、四川等地。

本草始载：始载于东汉《神农本草经》。

功效：疏散风热，疏肝解郁，升阳举陷。

主治：治疗感冒发热，肝郁气滞，月经不调，气虚下陷导致的脱肛及子宫下垂、胃下垂等。

Basic knowledge

Origin: The dry root of *Bupleurum chinensis* DC. or *B. scorzonerifolium* Willd. belonging to the family Umbelliferae. The former is called "Bei / North Chaihu", and the latter is called "Nan / South Chaihu."

Location: Bei Chaihu is mainly produced in Northeast China and North China; Nan Chaihu is mainly produced in Hubei Province and Sichuan Province.

First recorded in: *Shennong's Classic of Materia Medica* of the Eastern Han Dynasty.

Efficacy: Dispelling wind and heat, soothing liver and relieving depression, ascending up spleen-qi and yang.

Indications: Chaihu can treat cold and fever, liver depression with qi stagnation, irregular menstruation, rectal prolapse, uterine prolapse and gastroptosis due to sinking of middle qi.

拓展模块

柴胡是一味常用中药，应用于多种解表散热的中成药中，如小柴胡颗粒、小儿柴桂退热颗粒等。小柴胡汤是医圣张仲景《伤寒论》中记载的经典药方。但是，要注意的是，大家在使用这些中成药或经典药方时不能滥用，应当辩证对症才行。

生活中也可以用柴胡进行食疗，在煮粥、炖肉或炖鸡时可以加入少量柴胡，搭配不同的药材，能起到不同的保健作用。

Related information

Chaihu is a commonly used Chinese herbal medicine. It is applied in many kinds of Chinese patent medicines which can release exterior and cure fever, such as Xiaochaihu Keli, Xiao'er Chaigui Tuire Keli and so on. "Xiao Chaihu Tang" is one of the classic prescriptions recorded in *Treatise on Cold Pathogenic*, a medical classic written by Zhang Zhongjing, the Medical Sage. But it should be noted that you need to find out whether these patent medicines or the famous prescriptions are suitable for you when you want to use them to treat diseases.

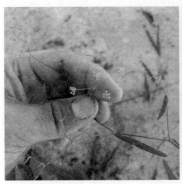 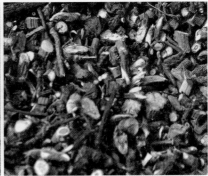

Chaihu can also be used for health care in daily life. When cooking porridge and stewing meat or chicken, you can add a small amount of Chaihu with different medicinal materials, and this will do good to your health.

故事模块

相传从前，一个黑心地主家里有两位长工，一位姓柴，一位姓胡。有一天姓胡的病了，地主不愿给他治病，便把姓胡的赶出了家门，姓柴的一气之下也离开了地主家。他二人便开始逃荒，在一座山中，姓胡的躺在地上走不动了，姓柴的便去给他找吃的。姓胡的肚子实在饿了，无意中拔了身边的一种草根充饥，居然把病治好了。从此，他们便用这种草为人治病，并以他二人的姓氏给这种草命名为"柴胡"。

这只是一个传说而已。但柴胡确实是自古至今历代医家常用的一味重要药材。清代名医陈平伯擅长用柴胡治病并此以闻名，他把《伤寒论》中的"小柴胡汤"，变换了2000多个方子，每张方子都有柴胡。

古典名著《红楼梦》的作者曹雪芹博学多闻，深谙中医之道。比如，在《红楼梦》第八十三回中描述了林黛玉生病的故事。林黛玉梦见她被

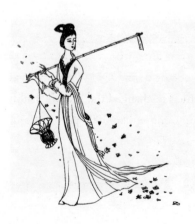

许配给他人续弦，宝玉手持小刀要挖出自己的心来向她表明真心，这时黛玉猛地从噩梦中惊醒，痰血上涌，一病不起。王太医为她诊脉后，一针见血地指出林黛玉的病是由于她平日郁结所致，伴有头晕、不思饮食、多梦易醒和多疑多惧的症状，需用柴胡配当归、白芍等药。贾宝玉的堂兄贾琏看过处方后质疑方子中的柴胡，王太医解释说：黛玉因

积郁致病，非柴胡不足以疏肝解郁，柴胡虽有升提阳气的作用，为吐血等病所忌，但用鳖血拌炒炮制即可。果不其然，黛玉服药后病情好转。

柴胡在战争中也起到过重要的作用。1939 年，太行山地区八路军战士受到日军和国民党部队双重封锁，当时抗战的很多八路军将士患上了流感、疟疾，高热不退，但由于受到封锁无药可用。时任 129 师卫生部长的钱信忠召集人员上山采集柴胡熬成汤药给病号服用，颇有效果。

Story

It is said that once upon a time, a black-hearted landlord had two long-term farm laborers, one had the surname Chai, and the other's surname was Hu. One day, Hu was ill seriously. The landlord did not want to spend money in treating him, so he drove Hu away. Out of indignation, Chai also left the landlord. So they set off on their journey together. When they were in a mountain, Hu was too tired and hungry to move, so he laid on the ground. Then Chai went away to look for food. As Hu was starving, he accidentally pulled out a kind of grass root beside him and ate some of the grass root. Out of his expectancy, he was cured by this root. Then the two began to use the herb to cure many people and named it Chaihu with their surnames.

The above story is just a legend. But Chaihu is an important medicinal herb commonly used by physicians from ancient times to the present. Chen Pingbo, a famous doctor in the Qing Dynasty, was famous for treating diseases with Chaihu. He changed the "Xiao Chaihu Tang" in *Treatise on Febrile Diseases* into more than 2000 prescriptions, and all of these prescriptions had Chaihu in them.

Cao Xueqin, the author of the classical novel *A Dream of Red Mansions*, was knowledgeable and good at TCM. For example, in the eighty-third chapter of this book, the story of Lin Daiyu's illness is described. Lin Daiyu dreamed that she would be married to a widow, and her lover Jia Baoyu cut himself on the chest in order to dig his heart out to show his true love to her. Lin Daiyu suddenly woke up from the nightmare, and became seriously ill. She coughed much phlegm with blood. Imperial plysician. Wang, an imperial physician, was assigned to treat her. After checking her pulse, Dr. Wang pointed out that Lin Daiyu's illness was caused by her daily depression, with syndromes such as dizziness, lack of appetite, easy awakening, sentimentality and fear. He prescribed Chaihu with Dang Gui, Bai Shao and so on. Jia Baoyu's cousin Jia Lian didn't agree with Chaihu in the prescription after reading it. Dr. Wang explained that Lin Daiyu was ill because of depression, and Chaihu was the best medicine to soothe liver and relieve depression. Though Chaihu had the function of promoting yang qi and was taboo for hematemesis, it still could be used if stir-fried with soft-shelled turtle blood. Sure enough, Lin Daiyu's condition improved after she took the medicine.

Chaihu also played an important role in the war. In 1939, the Eighth Route Army soldiers in Taihang Mountains were besieged by both Japanese and Kuomintang forces. At that time, many of these soldiers suffered from influenza and malaria, but there was no medicine available because of the siege. Qian Xinzhong, then Minister of Health of 129 Division, summoned soldiers to collect Chaihu in the mountains, and made Chaihu decoction for ill soldiers to take. This herb turned out to be very effective.

党参

Dangshen / Tangshen / Radix Codonopsis

知识模块

来源： 桔梗科（Campanulaceae）植物党参 *Codonopsis pilosula* (Franch.) Nannf.、素花党参 *C. pilosula* Nannf. var. *modesta* (Nannf.) L. T. Shen、川党参 *C. tangshen* Oliv. 的根。

产地： 山西、河南、陕西、甘肃、四川及东北地区。

本草始载： 始载于清代《本草从新》。

功效： 补脾益气，补血，生津。

主治： 治疗脾肺气虚证、气血两虚证，以及气短口渴等。

Basic knowledge

Origin: The root of *Codonopsis pilosula* (Franch.) Nannf., *C. pilosula* Nannf. var. *modesta* (Nannf.) L. T. Shen, or *C. tangshen* Oliv. belonging to the family Campanulaceae.

Location: Dangshen is mainly produced in Shanxi, Henan, Shaanxi, Gansu and Sichuan provinces, and Northeast China.

First recorded in: *Ben Cao Cong Xin* (*New Compilation of Materia Medica*) of the Qing dynasty

Efficacy: Invigorating spleen and replenishing qi, nourishing blood, promoting the generation of body fluid.

Indications: Dangshen can treat syndrome of lung-spleen qi deficiency, syndrome of both qi and blood deficiency, shortness of breath, thirst.

党参具有补血益气，健脾益肺的功效，而且价格便宜，是常用的传统补益药。在临床上，常用于治疗脾肺虚弱，气短心悸，食少便溏，虚喘咳嗽等症。党参被列入《可用于保健食品的物品名单》，生活中可以用党参泡茶、煮粥、炖汤，如党参乌鸡汤，能起到很好的养生保健作用。需要注意的是，党参不宜与藜芦同用。

购买党参时应该怎样挑选呢？党参最大的特征就是根头部的疣状突起，是它的茎痕和芽，看起来像极了中国传统石狮子雕塑头上的"卷发"，因此俗称"狮子头"或"狮子盘头"。质量好的党参切面外围是淡棕色，中间是淡黄色，形似菊花心。

Related information

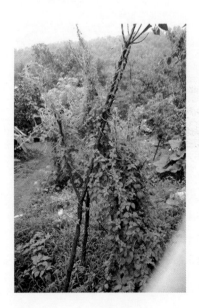

Dangshen has the effect of nourishing blood and replenishing qi, and invigorating the spleen and lung. Also its price is not high. Therefore, it is a commonly used traditional tonic medicine. In clinic, it is often used to treat spleen and lung weakness, shortness of breath, palpitation, loss of appetite, loose stool, asthma and cough. Dangshen is included in List of Items That Can Be Used as Health Food. In daily life, Dangshen can be made into tea, porridge and soup, such as Dangshen-silkie soup, which is

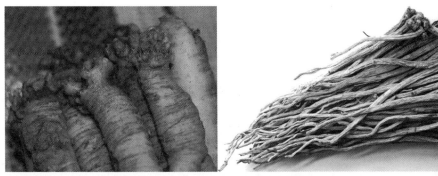

根茎上的疣状突起，在中药材上叫"狮子头"，它们都是茎痕及芽。

beneficial for health care. It should be noted that Dangshen cannot be used with Lilu (falsehellebore root and rhizome).

How do we select Dangshen with good quality? The biggest characteristic of Dangshen is the verrucous protuberances of the root head, which are its stem scars and buds, commonly known as "Shi Zi Tou" or "Shi Zi Pan Tou" (which means lion head) because they look like the "curly hair" on the head of traditional Chinese stone lions. The cut surface of good Dangshen is light brown in the periphery and light yellow in the middle, which resembles the center of chrysanthemum flowers.

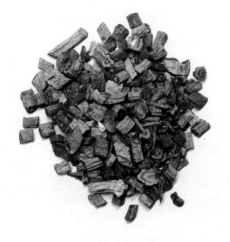

故事模块

药界流传这样一句谚语："千斤参，万斤参，不如黄松背的一棵五花芯。""五花芯"是山西省陵川县黄松背一带所产的一个名贵党参品种。切开参体后，断面纹路像盛开的五瓣花一样，所以起名叫"五花芯"。陵川县内一直流传着一个关于"花芯姑娘"的故事。

传说，在古时候，黄松背地区流传着一种疾病，人们不想吃饭，日夜咳喘，身上无力，田里的庄稼也荒废了。村里有户人家养了五个女儿，依次叫大花、二花、三花、四花、五花。她们父母早亡，从小跟着爷爷在山上采药，略懂一些药性和医道。五姐妹眼看着爷爷和乡亲们卧病在床，决心去寻访名医。

她们翻山越岭，走了三天三夜来到王莽岭的深山峡谷中，遇到了一位须发全白已经病入膏肓的采药老人。她们向老人请教，老人交给她们一包药材，然后断断续续告诉她们："一半阴、一半阳；放罢炮、挂铃铛；晚上握、白天凉；一出世、救苍生。"刚刚说完就去世了。

五姐妹急忙把药材带回村中熬煮，家人和乡亲们喝了，顿时感觉神清气爽，体力大增，纷纷开始下地干活，村子里又重现了往日的生机。原来这种植物就是党参。在之后的几年里，五位姑娘根据老人的教导，慢慢懂得了党参的得来之法。而且，经她们之手种出的党参切断后都是五个花瓣的形状，于是便产生了"五花芯"。

Story

In the TCM field, a proverb goes, "Even a thousand or ten thousand jin (1 jin equals 500 grams) of Renshen is not as precious as a Wu Hua Xin". "Wu Hua Xin" is a valuable type of Dangshen produced in the Huangsongbei area of Lingchuan County of Shanxi Province. If you cut it open, you will see the texture of the cross-section looks like a five-petal flower in full bloom, so it is called "Wu Hua Xin" (five-petal-flower). There is a story about this in Lingchuan County.

Legend has it that, in ancient times, a disease struck the Huangsongbei area. People didn't have any appetite, coughing day and night, and they became weaker and weaker, so the crops in the fields were abandoned. In a family of this village, there were five daughters, who were named Dahua, Erhua, Sanhua, Sihua and Wuhua (their names literally mean the big flower, the second flower, the third flower, the fourth flower and the fifth flower respectively). Their parents passed away early, and they always went to mountains to collect medicinal herbs with their grandfather. When the five sisters saw that their grandfather and other villagers were sick in bed, they were determined to go out to search for a famous doctor.

They climbed over the mountains and walked for three days and nights to the deep mountains named Wangmangling. There, they met a white-haired old man who also worked as a medicinal herb collector. The old man was suffering a serious disease that couldn't be cured. Hearing what they were looking for, the old man gave them a pack of herbs, and then told them in a weak voice, "Half yin, half yang; after the cracking sound, the bells hang; rub at night, air-cool in daylight; when coming out, it saves the life." Then the old man passed away.

The five sisters hurriedly took the medicine back to the village and prepared it for the fellow villagers. After drinking it, they soon felt refreshed and physically strong, and began to go to work in the fields. This herb turned out to be Dangshen. In the following years, the five girls slowly learned the way to cultivate and process this medicinal herb according to the instructions given by the old man. Moreover, the Dangshen planted by the five girls all showed the five-petal-flower picture when cut open, thus it got the name "Wu Hua Xin".

黄芩

Huangqin / Baical Skullcap Root / Radix Scutellariae

知识模块

来源： 唇形科（Labiatae）植物黄芩 *Scutellaria baicalensis* Georgi 的干燥根。

产地： 主产于河北、山西、内蒙古、辽宁等地。

本草始载： 始载于东汉《神农本草经》。

功效： 清热燥湿，泻火解毒，止血安胎。

主治： 治疗湿热引起的胸闷呕恶，湿热痢疾、黄疸，肺热咳嗽，疮痈肿毒，胎动不安。

Basic knowledge

Origin: The dry root of *Scutellaria baicalensis* Georgi belonging to the family Labiatae.

Location: Huangqin is mainly produced in Hebei Province, Shanxi Province, Inner Mongolian Autonomous Region, and Liaoning Province, etc.

First recorded in: *Shennong's Classic of Materia Medica* of the Eastern Han Dynasty.

Efficacy: Clearing heat and eliminating dampness, purging fire and relieving toxicity, stopping bleeding and preventing miscarriage.

Indications: Oppression in chest, vomiting and nausea due to damp-heat, dysentery, jaundice, cough due to lung heat, sore and abscesses, threatened abortion.

拓展模块

生活中也可用黄芩进行养生保健。如黄芩茶和黄芩粥。取黄芩 6 克，绿茶 3 克，黄芩用适量水煎沸后取汁用来冲泡绿茶，可以起到清热除烦、降压利尿作用。取黄芩、柴胡各 10 克，大米 50 克，先将黄芩、柴胡水煎取汁，然后加大米煮粥，最后加适量砂糖调味即可，对发热头痛、全身酸痛有明显疗效。但黄芩苦寒伤胃，脾胃虚寒者不宜使用。

Related information

Huangqin can also be used for health care in life. For example, Huangqin tea and Huangqin porridge are healthy for people. You can take 6 grams of Huangqin and 3 grams of green tea. Firstly boil Huangqin in water; then brew the green tea with this water. This tea can clear heat, relieve irritation, reduce blood pressure and induce diuresis. You can also take 10 grams of Huangqin, 10 grams of Chaihu, and 50 grams of rice. Boil Huangqin and Chaihu in water, and use the water to make porridge. Finally you can add some sugar to flavor the

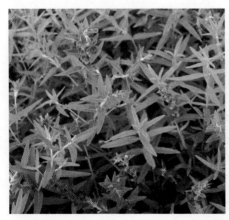
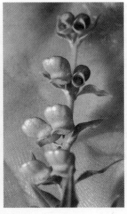

花萼形态很奇特，像帽子一样。花萼中可以看到小坚果。

103

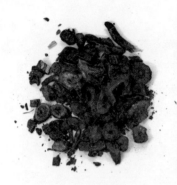
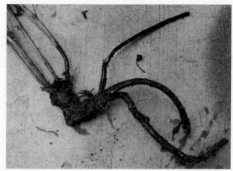

porridge. This porridge has obvious curative effect on fever, headache and general soreness of human body. However, Huangqin is bitter in taste and cold in nature, which is harmful for stomach. Therefore, those with deficiency cold of spleen and stomach had better not take it.

✎ 故事模块

我国的著名医药学家李时珍在《本草纲目》中记载了他的一次亲身经历。

在他 20 岁的时候，李时珍日夜苦读，全力以赴准备科举考试，却不小心染上了感冒咳嗽，可是李时珍并未在意。结果时间长了他总感到浑身发热，犹如火燎一般，而且久咳不止，总是咳出很多痰来。病情拖到夏天，更是感到烦热口渴，寝食难安。他尝试了多种中药，却丝毫不见好转，反而越来越厉害，为他诊病的郎中们都认为他的病无药可救了。李时珍的父亲李言闻也是位医生，他遍查医书，突然想起来名医李东垣的一个药方，于是就照着药方用黄芩一两，加两碗水煎成一碗给李时珍服下，结果李时珍很快就康复了。

通过这次的经历，李时珍深感中国医药学的神奇。他赞叹道："药中肯綮，如鼓应桴，医中之妙，有如此哉。"意为把药用到最关键的地方，就像用鼓槌去敲鼓一样，立即见效。

Story

Li Shizhen, a master of Chinese herbal medicine, recorded one of his personal experiences in his *Compendium of Materia Medica*.

When he was 20 years old, he studied hard day and night to prepare for the imperial examination. Accidentally he got cold and coughed a lot, but Li Shizhen did not care at first. After a period of time, he felt being burnt all over his body, and couldn't stop coughing up much phlegm. Even in the summer, he didn't get recovered, but felt more and more irritated and thirsty. He tried many kinds of Chinese herbal medicines, but they did not improve his condition at all. Instead, his disease became more and more severe. The doctors who treated him all said that the disease was incurable. Li Shizhen's father Li Yanwen was also a doctor. He looked through the medical books and suddenly recalled a prescription of a famous doctor named Li Dongyuan. Then, following this prescription, he decocted 50 grams of Huangqin in two bowls of water for Li Shizhen. Luckily, Li Shizhen recovered quickly after taking it.

Through this event, Li Shizhen was amazed by the miraculous effect of TCM. He praised it in this way: "How amazing the Traditional Chinese Medicine is! If you apply the right medicine to treat diseases, you will get the quickest effect, as quickly as you hear the sound when beating the drum with a drumstick."

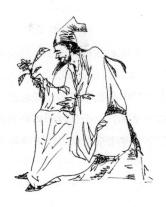

黄芪

Huangqi / Milkvetch Root / Radix Astragali seu Hedysari

来源：豆科（Leguminosae）植物蒙古黄芪 *Astragalus membranaceus* (Fisch.) Bge. var. *mongolicus* (Bge.) Hsiao 或膜荚黄芪 *A. membranaceus* (Fisch.) Bge. 的干燥根。

产地：产于内蒙古、山西及黑龙江等地。

本草始载：始载于东汉《神农本草经》。

功效：补气升阳，益卫固表，利水消肿，排脓，敛疮生肌。

主治：治疗气虚乏力，食少便溏，自汗，气虚水肿，疮疡久溃不敛等。

Basic knowledge

Origin: The dry root of *Astragalus membranaceus* (Fisch.) Bge. var. *mongolicus* (Bge.) Hsiao, or *A. membranaceus* (Fisch.) Bge. belonging to the family Leguminosae.

Location: Huangqi is mainly produced in Inner Mongolia Autonomous Region, Shanxi Province and Heilongjiang Province.

First recorded in: *Shennong's Classic of Materia Medica* of the Eastern Han Dynasty.

Efficacy: Tonifying qi and rasing yang, invigorating qi for consolidating superficies,inducing diuresis for removing edema, expelling pus healing sore and promoting granulation.

Indications: Qi deficiency and fatigue, poor appetite, loose stool, spontaneous sweating, edema due to deficiency of qi, sores and ulcers incurable after bursting.

拓展模块

　　黄芪是传统补气药，被称为"补气之王"。黄芪中富含黄芪多糖等物质，可用于提高机体免疫力，抗肿瘤，还能降血脂血糖、保护心脏。因此作为一味常用中药，黄芪对人体多有益处，而且黄芪被列入《可用于保健食品的物品名单》，在日常饮食中可以很方便地利用黄芪来补益身体。可以经常用黄芪泡水喝，比如黄芪和党参、茯苓煎水服用，能治疗脾虚；用黄芪和枸杞子煎水服用，有利于改善气血虚弱。黄芪也可以用来煮粥或炖汤，比如黄芪鸡肉粥、黄芪乌鸡汤、黄芪羊肉汤等，既美味又滋补。

Related information

Huangqi is a Chinese herbal medicine that is often used to invigorate qi, and it is called the "king of qi-invigorating medicines". Huangqi is rich in Astragalus polysaccharide, and can be used widely to improve immunity, prevent cancer, lower blood lipid and sugar, and protect heart. As a commonly used Chinese medicine, Huangqi is beneficial to human body. It is included in List of Items That Can Be Used as Health Food. In daily diet, Huangqi can be conveniently used to nourish the body. People can often drink tea made with Huangqi, such as water boiled with Huangqi, Dangshen and Fuling (poria) can be effective on spleen deficiency while water boiled with Huangqi and Gouqizi (Chinese wolfberry fruit) is good for qi and blood deficiency. Huangqi can also be used to cook porridge or stew soup, such as Huangqi-chicken porridge, Huangqi-silkie soup and Huangqi-mutton soup, which are both delicious and nourishing.

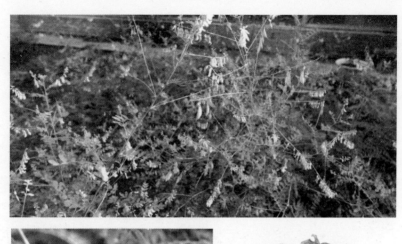

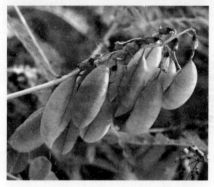
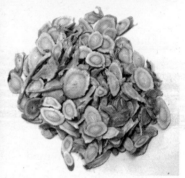

故事模块

　　黄芪的芪字，在古代写作"耆"，指的是六十岁的老人。黄芪在古代也写作"黄耆"。李时珍在《本草纲目》中解释了这个耆字："耆，长也，黄耆色黄，为补药之长，故名。"

　　黄芪最早记载在《神农本草经》，叫"戴糁"，相传是为了纪念一个名叫戴糁的人。相传戴糁是一位善良的老中医，一生乐于救助他人。一天老人上山采药，路过一处悬崖，只听有妇人在悬崖边哭喊求救，原来妇人的孩子不小心掉下了悬崖，所幸被一棵小树勾住，正倒挂在悬崖上。老人连忙放下药篓，小心翼翼地顺着悬崖爬下去，托起小孩，又慢慢地把小孩送到妇人手中。就在孩子成功脱险的刹那，老人脚底一空，不幸坠下了悬崖。

人们在悬崖下找到老人的遗体，并将其安葬。后来老人的墓旁长了一种草药，有补气之效，治好了很多人的病。为了纪念老人，人们便将这种药命名为"戴糁"。由于老人身形消瘦，面色淡黄，人们称他为"黄耆"以示尊敬。于是人们也将这种草药称为"黄耆"，后来改为"黄芪"。

虽然这只是一个民间传说故事，但是老人这种奋不顾身救下幼童的勇气和行为，值得所有人的敬佩，也体现出医者仁心厚德治病救人的高尚精神。

Story

The Chinese name of Huangqi is 黄芪. In ancient times, "芪" was written as "耆" which refers to the 60-year-old men. So "黄芪" was also written as "黄耆". Li Shizhen explained this Chinese character in *Compendium of Materia Medica*, "耆 means the elderly; 黄耆 got its name because it is yellow ("黄" means yellow) and also because it is the best among the tonic medicines."

Huangqi was first recorded in *Shennong's Classic of Materia Medica*, and it was called "Daishen". It is said that the name was to commemorate a person named Dai Shen. According to legend, Dai Shen was a kind-hearted old Chinese doctor who was willing to help others all his life. One day the old man went up to the mountain to collect medicinal herbs, he heard a woman crying for help at the edge of the cliff. It turned out the woman's child fell off the cliff. Luckily he was caught by a small tree, and was hanging upside down there. Seeing the boy was in extreme danger, the old man immediately put down the medicine basket, carefully climbed down the cliff, caught the child and slowly delivered him to the woman. Unfortunately, when the child succeeded in escaping from danger, the old man slipped and fell off the cliff and died.

People found his body under the cliff and buried him. Later, a kind of herb grew beside his grave. This herb had the effect of invigorating qi, and cured many people. In order to commemorate the old man, people named this herb "Daishen" after him. The old man was thin and had a pale yellow complexion, and people called him "Huang Qi/黄耆" (which literally means "yellow old man") to show respect. So people also named this herb "黄耆" and later changed it to "黄芪".

Although this is only a folklore story, the courage and behavior of the elderly man to save the young children even at the cost of his own life deserve the respect of all people. The story also reflects the benevolence, kindness and morality of good doctors.

黄连
Huanglian / Rhizome of Chinese Goldthread / Rhizoma Coptidis

来源：毛茛科（Ranunculaceae）植物黄连 *Coptis chinensis* Franch.、三角叶黄连 *C. deltoidea* C.Y. Cheng et Hsiao 或云连 *C. teeta* Wall. 的干燥根茎。

产地：产于重庆、湖北及云南等地。

本草始载：始载于东汉《神农本草经》。

功效：清热燥湿，泻火解毒。

主治：治疗各种湿热证及热毒证。

Basic knowledge

Origin: The dry rhizome of *Coptis chinensis* Franch., *C. deltoidea* C.Y. Cheng et Hsiao or *C. teeta* Wall. belonging to the family Ranunculaceae.

Location: Huanglian is mainly produced in Chongqing city, Hubei province and Yunnan province, etc.

First recorded in: *Shennong's Classic of Materia Medica* of the Eastern Han Dynasty.

Efficacy: Clearing heat and drying dampness, purging fire and relieving toxicity.

Indications: Various damp-heat syndrome and heat-toxin syndrome.

提到黄连，你或许会想起"哑巴吃黄连，有苦说不出"这句歇后语。确实，黄连极苦，但它确是一味良药，能够清热燥湿，泻火解毒，可治疗温热呕吐、泻痢、黄疸、湿疹、咽喉肿痛等，也可降血压、降血糖等。黄连的提取物黄连素，常用于抗炎和抗腹泻药物。但要注意，黄连大苦大寒，因此胃寒呕吐、脾虚泄泻等患者忌用。

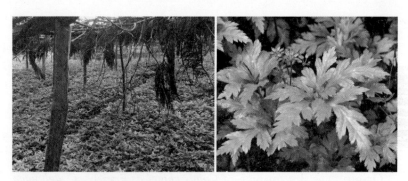

黄连属喜阴植物，需要搭棚种植

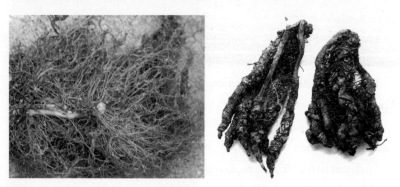

刚挖出来的黄连。黄连根茎和不定根的颜色，非常鲜黄，这都是黄连中有效成分黄连素，又称小檗碱的颜色。

Speaking of Huanglian, you might think of the famous Chinese saying: "When the dumb man eats the bitter herb Huanglian, he has to suffer in silence." It is true that Huanglian is extremely bitter, but it is also a good medicine, which can clear away heat, dry dampness, purge fire and clear toxicity. It can treat vomiting due to damp-heat, diarrhea, jaundice, eczema, sore throat, and so on. It can also reduce blood pressure and blood sugar. Berberine extracted from Huanglian is often used in anti-inflammatory and anti-diarrhea medicines. But it needs to be noted that Huanglian is extremely bitter in taste and rather cold in nature, so patients with vomiting due to cold stomach and diarrhea due to spleen deficiency should not use it.

故事模块

相传很久以前，在重庆石柱县住着一位姓陶的大夫，和女儿相依为命。由于陶大夫经常要外出替人诊病，于是就雇了一位名叫黄连的帮工为他种花栽药。

有一年春天，陶大夫的女儿外出踏青，看见郊外山上长着一种开绿色小花的小草，十分喜欢，便顺手拔了几棵带回家种在园子里。黄连每次照顾药草时便一同照料着这几棵小草，在他的精心照料下，这种植物长得越来越茂盛。

次年夏天，陶大夫外出给人治病，要许久不能回家，但是他的女儿突然患病卧床，浑身燥热，又吐又拉，一天天消瘦下去。陶大夫的几位朋友想尽一切办法也没能治好小姑娘的病。

这时候，黄连突然想到了种在园子里的那种小草，他曾经用这种小草治好了自己的嗓子痛，会不会对陶大夫女儿的病也能见效？于是他便从园中拔下这种草来煎药，让小姑娘喝下。没多久，小姑娘的病竟然痊愈了。

　　陶大夫回来后，问明白了来龙去脉，便连声感谢黄连说："小女患的是肠胃湿热，一定要清热燥湿的药才医得好。看来，这种小草有很好的清热燥湿功效啊！"为了感谢帮工黄连，这药材也就取名为黄连。时至今日，石柱县仍然是黄连的主产区。

Story

It is said that a long time ago, a doctor with surname Tao lived with his only daughter in Shizhu County of Chongqing. The doctor often went out to see the patients, so he hired a man named Huang Lian to plant flowers and herbs for him.

One spring, the doctor's daughter went for an outing. She noticed a grass with small green flowers. She liked the flowers very much, so she took some of the grass back home and planted them in the garden. Huang Lian would take care of these grasses when he was working in the garden. The grasses gradually flourished thanks to his care.

The following summer, the doctor went out to treat patients for a period of time. During that period, his daughter suddenly fell ill with the symptoms of fever, vomiting and diarrhea. She turned thinner gradually. Several friends of the doctor tried every means to treat her, but all of them failed to cure the girl's illness.

Then, Huang Lian recalled that he had once cured his sore throat with the grasses in the garden, and he wondered whether this herb could save the doctor's daughter. So he picked some of this herb from the garden and boiled it in water. Then he asked the little girl to drink the soup. Not long after taking it, the girl's illness was cured. After the doctor came back, his family told him what had happened. He then thanked the helper and said, "My daughter was suffering from gastrointestinal heat and dampness. The disease can only be cured by medicines with efficacy of clearing heat and drying dampness. It seems this grass is just the one for this!" Because the helper was called Huang Lian, in order to thank him, this medicine was named after him. From then on, Shizhu County has always been the main producing area of Huanglian.

葛根

Gegen / Lobed Kudzuvine Root / Radix Puerariae

来源： 豆科（Leguminosae）植物野葛 *Pueraria lobata* (Willd.) Ohwi 的干燥根。

产地： 主产于湖南、河南、广东等地。

本草始载： 始载于东汉《神农本草经》。

功效： 疏散退热，透疹，生津，升阳止泻。

主治： 外感发热头痛，口渴，麻疹不透，泄泻以及心血管疾病等。

Basic knowledge

Origin: The dry root of *Pueraria lobata* (willd.) Ohwi. belonging to the family Leguminosae.

Location: Gegen is mainly produced in Hunan, Henan, and Guangdong provinces, etc.

First recorded in: *Shennong's Classic of Materia Medica* of the Eastern Han Dynasty.

Efficacy: Releasing exterior and curing fever, promoting eruption, promoting the production of body fluid, ascending yang to stop diarrhea.

Indications: High fever of exterior syndromes, thirst, measles without adequate eruption, diarrhea, cardiovascular disease, etc.

拓展模块

葛根具有扩张血管、降糖降脂的作用，特别适用于经常饮酒吸烟的人，以及高血压、高血脂、高血糖及偏头痛等心脑血管病患者等。葛花也是一味中药，能解酒醒脾，适用于醉酒和酒精中毒。

但是这里所说的葛根与大家在市场上买的葛根粉可不是一回事。这里的葛根是豆科植物野葛的块根，药用价值更高。而食用的葛根粉来源于粉葛，即豆科植物甘葛藤的干燥根，粉葛可药食两用，但它的淀粉含量高，更多用于加工淀粉食用，制成葛粉、葛根茶、葛根粉丝等多种产品，是良好的保健食品。

Related information

Gegen has the functions of dilating blood vessels, and lowering blood sugar and blood lipid. Therefore, it is especially suitable for people who often drink alcohol and smoke cigarettes, as well as the patients with cardia-cerebrovascular diseases with symptoms such as hypertension, hyperlipidemia, hyperglycemia and migraine, etc. Flower of Gegen is also a medicine which can relieve alcoholism and refresh the mind. It is suitable for alcohol intoxication.

But the Gegen mentioned here is not the same as the Gegen powder commonly seen in the market. Gegen here is the root tuber of a plant named Yege (*Pueraria lobata* (Willd.) Ohwi), and it has higher medicinal value. Edible Gegen powder comes from Fenge, the tuber of a plant named Gangeteng (*Pueraria thomsonii* Benth.). Fenge can be used for both medicine and food. But it is rich in starch, and is more often processed to get starch for food, such as Gegen powder, Gegen tea, Gegen silk noodles which are good health food.

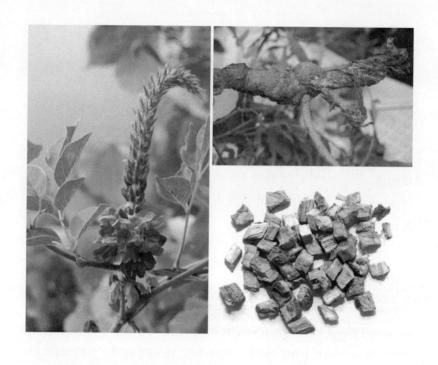

故事模块

　　相传，古时候在一处深山密林中住着一位白发苍苍的老人，以挖药卖药为生。

　　有一天，他正采药时，一个十来岁的男孩急匆匆跑到他面前求救："老爷爷，快救救我吧！"老人连忙问他缘由。原来，孩子的父亲是远近闻名的葛员外。葛员外为人正直，得罪了朝中权贵，遭到恶人诬告"密谋造反"。可恶的昏君信以为真，便派人对葛家满门抄斩，只有这个孩子逃了出来，不料却被官兵发现，因此一路逃亡至此。

　　善良的老人动了恻隐之心，于是拉起孩子就往深山密林里钻，把孩子带到一个非常隐秘的山洞里。官兵们在山上搜索了好长时间，一直没见着孩子的影子，就只好收兵回去了。直到这时，老人才带着孩子从山洞里走出来。

　　老人让孩子自己去找个容身之地，可是孩子却跪下来对老人苦苦哀求："我全家被满门抄斩，我已经无家可归了。请您收留我吧。我不怕吃苦，愿意跟着您学本领。"老人非常同情这个男孩，就把他留在了自己身边，每天带着他去山中采药。时间长了，通过向老人学习，孩子认识了很多草药，尤其对一种色白肥大而坚实的草根印象最深。这种草根能治疗发热、口渴、腹泻等疾病。

　　后来，老人过世了，孩子也长大了，他用这种草根治好了不少病人。当人们问起草根的名字时，他不由想起了自己的身世和老人的救命之恩，便说道："这种药材叫作葛根。""葛"是他的姓氏，而"根"既表明这是一种草根，也寓意白发老人为葛家保存下了他这样一条"根"。

Story

According to legend, in ancient times, a white-haired old man lived in mountain forest, making his living by collecting and selling herbal medicines.

One day, while he was collecting medicinal herbs in the mountain, a teenage boy rushed to him and asked for help, "Grandpa. Please, please help me!" The old man asked the boy what had happened. It turned out that the child's father was a rich landowner with the surname Ge. Mr. Ge was a man of integrity, and had offended some powerful man in the royal court. Therefore, he was slandered by some villains for "treason". The stupid emperor believed the rumors, and sent his soldiers to kill the whole family of Mr. Ge. The child was the only one who escaped, but he was found and being chased by the soldiers.

The kind-hearted old man sympathized with the boy. He held the boy's hand and led him into the thick forest until they came into a secret cave. The soldiers searched for a long time but couldn't find the boy, so they left. Until now the old man and the boy dared to come out of the cave.

The old man asked the boy to leave and find a secure place himself. However, the boy knelt on his knees and said to the old man, "All my family members have been killed. I've lost my home. Please allow me to follow you. I'm not afraid of hardship. I want to learn skills from you." Sympathetic to the boy, the old man agreed. Thence, the old man took the child to the mountains every day to collect medicinal herbs. After a long time, by learning from the old man, the child gradually got to know a lot of herbs, especially a white-skinned, thick and solid grass root. This grass root can treat fever, thirst, diarrhea and other diseases.

After a few years, the old man passed away and the child grew up. He used this kind of grass root to cure many patients. When people asked him the name of the root, he couldn't help thinking of his own life and the life-saving grace of the old man. He said, "This medicine is called Ge Gen." "Ge" is his surname, and "Gen" which means "root" has two indications: first, this is a kind of grass root; second, the old man with white hair saved him and thus kept the "root" for the Ge family.

紫草

Zicao / Gromwell Root / Radix Arnebiae

知识模块

来源：紫草科（Boraginaceae）植物新疆紫草 *Arnebia euchroma* (Royle) Johnst.、内蒙古紫草 *A. guttata* Bunge. 或紫草 *Lithosperaum erythrorhizon* Sieb. et Zucc. 的干燥根。

产地：新疆紫草习称"软紫草"，主产于新疆、西藏；内蒙古紫草主产于内蒙古和甘肃。紫草习称"硬紫草"，主产于华北及东北。

本草始载：始载于东汉《神农本草经》。

功效：凉血活血，解毒透疹。

主治：治疗斑疹紫黑，麻疹不透，湿疹，疮疡，水火烫伤。

Basic knowledge

Origin: The dry root of *Arnebia euchroma* (Royle) Johnst., *A. guttata* Bunge., or *Lithosperaum erythrorhizon* Sieb. et Zucc. belonging to the family Boraginaceae.

Location: The first is called "Ruan / soft Zicao", and is mainly produced in Xinjiang Autonomous Region and Tibet Autonomous Region; the second is mainly produced in Inner Mongolia Autonomous Region and Gansu Province. The third is called "Ying / hard Zicao" and is mainly produced in North China and Northeast China.

First recorded in: *Shennong's Classic of Materia Medica* of the Eastern Han Dynasty.

Efficacy: Cooling blood and activating blood, removing toxicity and promoting eruption.

Indications: Macule in dark purple color, measles without adequate eruption, eczema, sores and ulcers, burn due to hot liquid or fire.

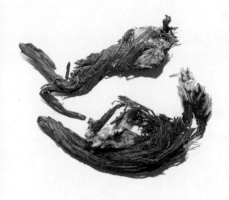
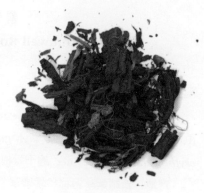

拓展模块

　　紫草外用治疗烧烫伤效果很好，紫草油外用可以治疗婴幼儿尿布疹。此外，紫草素也是一种天然色素，可以作为食品添加剂加入到食品中。

Related information

　　Zicao is very effective in treating burns caused by both fire and hot liquid when externally applied. Zicao oil can treat diaper rash of infants. In addition, alkannin extracted from Zicao is also a natural pigment that can be added to food as a food additive.

故事模块

　　紫草的花和根为什么是紫色的呢？据说这与一个凄美的爱情故事有关。

　　相传，一个偏远的小镇上住着一对相爱的夫妻。一天，妻子高热不退，昏睡不醒，身上起了许多紫黑色斑疹。他们看了很多郎中，用了许多药，病却迟迟不见好。丈夫愁肠百结，天天虔诚地拜佛祈祷，希望妻子能够早日醒来。一天天过去了，丈夫的膝盖都跪出了血，佛祖终于被他感动。

一日，他在冥冥之中听见佛问自己："你愿意用自己的生命来救她吗？"他毫不犹豫地答应了。佛接着说："这里有一棵草，你每天必须用自己的鲜血来浇灌它。等它开花时，你要用紫色花根熬水给你妻子喝，她的病自然就会好的。"

丈夫喜出望外，听从了佛祖的话，每天取自己的鲜血来浇灌这棵草，小心翼翼地照料它，盼望它早日开花。到了盛夏时节，这棵草终于开出了紫色的小花，丈夫激动地挖出了它紫色的根，煎熬汤水给妻子喝下。终于，妻子醒来了，而丈夫却因失血过多，带着幸福的微笑永远闭上了双眼。因为这种草的花和根都是紫色的，人们便称之为紫草。

Story

The flowers and roots of Zi Cao are purple. Why? It is said to be related to a tragic love story.

Legend has it that long time ago a loving couple lived in a remote town. One day, the wife got fever, and she was unconscious for a long time and could not be woken up. Besides, she had purplish-black rash on her skin. The husband took her to see many doctors, but none of the doctors could cure the disease. The husband was extremely worried and knelt down to pray to the Buddha devoutly every day, hoping that his wife could wake up as soon as possible. As the days passed, the husband's knees were bleeding, and the Buddha was finally touched by his faithfulness.

One day, he heard the Buddha ask him, "Would you like to save your wife at the cost of your own life?" He agreed without hesitation. The Buddha went on to say, "Here is a special grass. You must use your own blood to water it every day. When it blooms, you should dig out the purple roots, boil them and let your wife drink the soup. Her illness will be cured very soon."

123

The husband was overjoyed. Following the Buddha's words, he took his own blood every day to water the grass, and carefully took care of it, hoping that it would bloom soon. In the midsummer, the grass finally put forth purple flowers, and the husband excitedly dug out its purple roots and boiled the soup for his wife. Finally, his wife woke up, but he died with a happy smile because of excessive blood loss. Because the flowers and roots of this herb were purple, people called it Zicao (which literally means "purple grass").

（二）全草类 / Whole herb

广藿香
Guanghuoxiang / Cablin Patchouli Herb /
Herba Pogostemonis

知识模块

来源：唇形科（Labiatae）植物广藿香 *Pogostemon cablin* (Blanco) Benth. 的干燥地上部分。

产地：主产于海南、广东等地。一般认为广东石牌产的广藿香为道地药材。

本草始载：始载于东汉《异物志》。

功效：芳香化湿，开胃止呕，发表解暑。

主治：治疗湿阻中焦证，暑湿导致的腹泻呕吐等。

Basic knowledge

Origin: The dry aerial part of *Pogostemon cablin* (Blanco) Benth. belonging to the family Labiatae.

Location: Guanghuoxiang is mainly produced in Hainan and Guangdong provinces. Guanghuoxiang from Shipai, Guangdong Province is generally known as the genuine regional medicine.

First recorded in: *Yi Wu Zhi* (*Records of Foreign Matters*) of the Eastern Han Dynasty.

Efficacy: Resolving dampness with aromatics, increasing appetite and arresting vomiting, relieving exterior syndrome by diaphoresis, and clearing summer heat.

Indications: Syndrome of damp obstruction in middle energizer, diarrhea and vomiting caused by summer-heat and dampness.

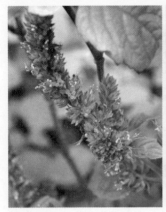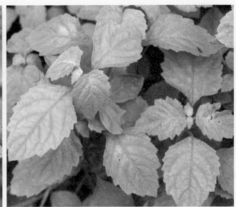

拓展模块

广藿香是我国著名南药之一，原产于菲律宾、马来西亚和印度等国。自宋代开始，广藿香就引入我国引种栽培，至今已有千年历史。

广藿香除药用外，其提取的精油香味浓郁而持久，是很好的定香剂，广泛用于香水中。此外，它被收录于《既是食品又是药品的物品名单》。因其具有健脾益气的功效，它也是一种不错的烹饪原料，它的嫩茎叶是野味之佳品，可凉拌、炒食和炸食，也可做粥。夏季可以用它来煮粥或泡茶饮用，可发表解暑，开胃止呕。人们常用的"藿香正气水"等中成药就是用广藿香提取出的广藿香油做主料制成的，常用来治疗感冒、呕吐、腹泻和中暑等症。

Related information

Guanghuoxiang is one of the famous medicines in Southern China. It originates from the Philippines, Malaysia, India and other countries. It has been one thousand years since Guanghuoxiang was introduced into China during the Song Dynasty.

Besides medicinal purposes, the essential oil extracted from it has a strong and persistent fragrance. Therefore, it is a good fixative agent and is widely used in perfumes. In addition, it is included in List of Items That Are both Food and Medicine. Since it has the effect of invigorating the spleen and invigorating qi, it is also a good cooking ingredient. Its tender stems and leaves are delicious, and can be served with sauce, or can be sautéed, fried, or made into porridge. In summer, porridge or tea made of Guanghuoxiang can help people relieve summer heat, increase appetite, and arrest vomiting. Some Chinese patent medicines such as "Huoxiang Zhengqi Shui" are commonly used by people to deal with cold, vomiting, diarrhea, sunstroke and so on. Their main ingredient is patchouli oil extracted from Guanghuoxiang.

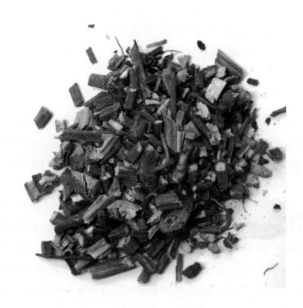

故事模块

很久以前，有一户人家，父母去世的早，只有哥哥和妹妹相依为命，妹妹有个好听的名字叫作霍香。后来，哥哥娶亲后就一直从军在外，留下姑嫂二人在家共同劳作，相互扶持。

一年夏天，天气十分闷热潮湿，霍香的嫂子因劳累过度而中暑晕倒，于是霍香就进山为嫂子采药，直到天黑时才提着一小筐药草回到家里。但是，霍香在采药时不慎被毒蛇咬伤，中了蛇毒。等乡亲们听见嫂子的呼救声，将郎中找来，却为时已晚，霍香已经中毒身亡。嫂子用霍香采来的药草治好了病。为了牢记霍香的恩情，嫂子便把这种有香味的药草称为"霍香"。从此"霍香"草的名声越传越广，治好了不少中暑的病人。因为是药草的缘故，人们在霍字头上加了一个"草"字头，将霍香写成了"藿香"。

这则民间传说故事里出现的正是中药"藿香"。但是，现在常用的药材为"广藿香"，藿香与广藿香功效相似，都是祛暑化湿、和胃止呕的常用中药材，但藿香的功效较广藿香要弱一些。"藿香正气水"等中成药里用到的主要成分即为广藿香油。

Story

Once upon a time, there was a family. In this family, the elder brother and the younger sister named Huo Xiang depended on each other. After the elder brother got married, he joined the army, leaving his wife and sister working together at home and supporting each other.

One summer, as the weather was extremely hot and humid, the wife of elder brother got sunstroke when she was working. Therefore, Huo Xiang went to the mountains to collect some medicinal herbs for her sister-in-law. It was already dark when she came home with a small basket of herbs. Unfortunately, Huo Xiang was bitten by a poisonous snake while she was looking for the medicine in the mountain. When the neighbors heard the call for help and sent for a doctor, it was too late, and Huo Xiang was already dead. The wife of the brother recovered after taking the herbs picked by Huo Xiang, and in order to memorize the kindness of Huo Xiang, she named this fragrant herb "霍香(Huoxiang)". Since then, this herb became well-known by the common people, and has cured many patients with sunstroke. Because it is a kind of herb, people add "艹" which is a sign of "grass" in Chinese to the head of "霍", and thus this special herb got its Chinese name "藿香".

This folklore tells the story of "Huoxiang", but nowadays "Guanghuoxiang" is a much more commonly used medicinal material. They are very similar. Actually Huoxiang and Guanghuoxiang are two similar Chinese medicines both for dispelling heat and dampness, and stopping vomiting. But the efficacy of Huoxiang is weaker than that of Guanghuoxiang. Patchouli oil extracted from Guanghuoxiang is the main ingredient used in some Chinese patent medicines such as Huoxiang Zhengqi Shui.

益母草
Yimucao / Motherwort Herb / Herba Leonuri

知识模块

来源：唇形科（Labiatae）植物益母草 *Leonurus japonicus* Houtt. 的地上部分。

产地：我国大部分地区均有产地。

本草始载：始载于东汉《神农本草经》。

功效：活血调经，利水消肿，清热解毒。

主治：治疗妇科痛经、经闭及产后瘀滞腹痛等瘀血证，以及水肿、小便不利等症。

Basic knowledge

Origin: The aerial part of *Leonurus japonicus* Houtt. belonging to the family Labiatae.

Location: Yimucao is mainly produced in most parts of China.

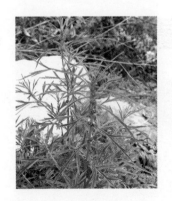

First recorded in: *Shennong's Classic of Materia Medica* of the Eastern Han Dynasty.

Efficacy: Activating blood and regulating menstruation, promoting diuresis and alleviating edema, clearing heat and relieving toxicity.

Indications: Dysmenorrhea, amenorrhea, blood stasis such as postpartum abdominal pain caused by stasis, edema and difficult urination.

拓展模块

本品为妇科调经要药，被收录于《可用于保健食品的物品名单》中。生活中可以用它进行食疗，如益母草茶、益母草炖乌鸡等，有助于治疗女性月经不调、痛经和不孕等。益母草果实为茺蔚子，亦是中药，能够清肝明目。

但益母草的作用不单单局限在治疗妇科病，它还可以用来美容，并治疗肾炎、水肿等疾病。比如，《新唐书》中记载武则天虽然年老，但由于她用一种特殊的药膏涂脸，所以看起来皮肤红润，根本看不出衰老。武则天去世四十多年后，王焘《外台秘要》专载武则天长期用过的一款外涂美容药方，其中的主要药物就是益母草。

Related information

Yimucao is an important medicine which is often used to regulate menstruation, and it is included in List of Items That Can Be Used as Health Food. It can be used in life to help keep healthy. For example, Yimucao herbal tea and stewed silkie with Yimucao can help treat irregular menstruation, dysmenorrhea and infertility, etc. Its fruit called as Chongweizi (motherwort fruit) is also a medicine which has the

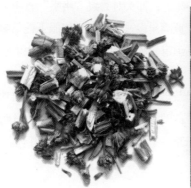
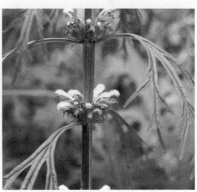

function of removing liver-fire for improving eyesight.

However, Yimucao is not only an important medicine for gynecological diseases, but also an ingredient in some beauty products. Besides, it is also often used to treat nephritis and edema, etc. According to *Xin Tang Shu* (*New History of the Tang Dynasty*), Wu Zetian, the only woman empress regnant in ancient China, often applied a special ointment on her face. Therefore, she looked healthy and didn't show any sign of senility even in her old age. Forty years after her death, Wang Tao of Tang Dynasty in his medical book named *Wai Tai Mi Yao* recorded the prescription of an externally applied cosmetic chronically used by Wu Zetian, and the main ingredient in it was Yimucao.

故事模块

相传古时候有一个名叫秀娘的女子，她心地十分善良。在她婚后不久，便怀了孕。一天，秀娘正在家中纺棉花，突然一只被猎人打伤了的黄麂跑过来，只见它双眼含泪，可怜巴巴地望着秀娘，请求她的帮助。秀娘见它十分可怜，就把它从猎人手中救了下来。不久之后，秀娘临盆，却不幸难产，十分危险。正当一家人束手无策时，门口传来不知什么动物"咯咯"的叫声。秀娘的丈夫打开门一看，正是秀娘救下的那只黄麂。只见它嘴里叼着一株药草来到秀娘的床前，仰头对秀娘"咯咯"直叫。秀娘猜到了它的来意，便叫丈夫从黄麂嘴里接过药草。秀娘服下香草煎的汤药后，疼痛渐渐地止住了，感到浑身轻松，没过多久便顺利生下了婴儿。因为这种草对女性大有益处，于是人们给它起名叫"益母草"。

当然，这只是个民间传说，但是益母草的名字确实是来源于它的功效，李时珍在《本草纲目》中记载着："（益母草）其功宜于妇人及明目益精，故有益母、益明之称。"益母草在《神农本草经》中被列为上品，是历代医家用来治疗妇科病的要药。

Story

According to legend, there was a woman named Xiuniang in ancient times. She was very kind-hearted. Shortly after her marriage, she was pregnant. One day, while Xiuniang was spinning cotton at home, suddenly, a muntjac wounded by a hunter came running up to her. It looked at Xiuniang with tears in its eyes, asking for help. Xiuniang saw that it was very pathetic and saved it from the hunter. Soon, she was giving birth to a baby, but unfortunately she had a difficult labor. Just when the family was worried and helpless, there came some strange sound of an animal. Xiuniang's husband opened the door and found that the sound came from the muntjac Xiuniang had rescued. With some grasses in his mouth, the muntjac came to Xiuniang, raised his head, and seemed to be saying something to Xiuniang. Immediately, Xiuniang got the meaning of the muntjac, and told her husband to take the grass from his mouth. After drinking the soup decocted with the grass, she felt relaxed, and gave birth to a baby soon after. Because this grass is of great benefit to women, people call it "Yi Mu Cao" which means "a grass beneficial for mothers".

Of course, this is only a story, but the name of Yimucao is really derived from its efficacy. Li Shizhen wrote in *Compendium of Materia Medica* that "(Yimucao) is good for women and beneficial for eyesight and essence, so it is called Yi Mu (which literally means beneficial for mothers) and Yi Ming (which literally means beneficial for eyesight)". It is listed as a top grade medicine in *Shennong's Classic of Materia Medica*, and it is an important medicine for gynecologic diseases used by doctors of all dynasties.

麻黄

Mahuang / Ephedra Herb / Herba Ephedrae

知识模块

来源： 麻黄科（Ephedraceae）植物草麻黄 *Ephedra sinica* Stapf、中麻黄 *E. intermedia* Schrenk et C. A. Mey. 或木贼麻黄 *E. equisetina* Bge. 的干燥草质茎。

产地： 产于我国三北地区。

本草始载： 始载于东汉《神农本草经》。

功效： 发汗解表，宣肺平喘，止咳，利尿消肿。

主治： 治疗风寒感冒，咳喘，水肿及小便不利等症。

Basic knowledge

Origin: The dry herbaceous stem of *Ephedra sinica* Stapf, *E. intermedia* Schrenk et C. A. Mey, or *E. equisetina* Bge. belonging to the family Ephedraceae.

Location: Mahuang is mainly produced in Northeast, Northwest and North of China.

First recorded in: *Shennong's Classic of Materia Medica* of the Eastern Han Dynasty.

Efficacy: Inducing sweating and releasing exterior, releasing stagnated lung-qi and relieving asthma, alleviating cough, promoting urination to reduce edema.

Indications: Wind-cold type common cold, cough and asthma, edema, and difficult urination.

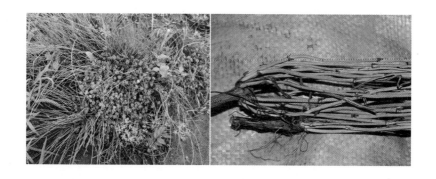

麻黄有较高的生态价值，麻黄地下根茎发达，适应性强，多分布在戈壁、沙漠等环境下，是优良的固沙植物，对保护生态环境具有不可替代的作用。此外，由于麻黄提取物麻黄碱是制造冰毒的原料，所以麻黄属于国家管制药材。

Related information

Mahuang has high ecological values. Its underground roots are well developed and highly adaptable to environment. Therefore, it is an excellent sand-fixating plant and plays an irreplaceable role in protecting the ecological environment in deserts. In addition, the ephedrine extracted from Mahuang can be used to produce methamphetamine which is also called as crystal meth, so it is one of the state controlled medicinal materials.

故事模块

从前，有个挖药的老人，无儿无女，他只收了一个徒弟。这个徒弟聪明伶俐，师傅很喜欢他，想把毕生所学都传授给他。但这个徒弟很是狂妄，刚刚学会一点皮毛，就以为自己很了不起了，根本不把师傅放在眼里。师傅伤透了心，就让徒弟另立门户，但在徒弟临走之前警告他说，有一种叫"无叶草"的药必须谨慎使用，因为这种草药的茎和根用处不同，发汗用茎，止汗用根，一旦弄错就会闹出人命。但是，徒弟却毫不在意，压根没把师傅的话放在心上。

从此，徒弟就离开了师傅另立门户，给人看病行医。可是，没过几天，徒弟就用无叶草治死了一个病人，被死者家属抓住去见官。县官经过审判，发现病人出虚汗，本应用麻黄根止汗，可是徒弟却错用麻黄的茎，他医术不精治死了人，便判他入狱三年。

经过这场牢狱之灾，徒弟明白了中医的博大精深，深刻地认识到自己的错误，非常懊悔。他出狱后找到师傅表示痛改前非。师傅见他有了转变，这才把他留下，继续向他传授医术。从此，徒弟再用"无叶草"时就十分谨慎小心了。因为这种草他惹过麻烦，就给它起名叫作"麻烦草"，后来又因为这草的根是黄色的，才又改叫"麻黄"。

虽说这只是个民间传说故事，但也表明医生给病人看病开药可容不得半点马虎，一旦用错药，就会造成严重的后果。医务工作是一件既严肃又神圣的工作，从医者必须要用耐心和细心去对待每一位患者。

Story

Once there was a childless old man who made a living by collecting medical herbs. He had an apprentice who was very smart. The old man decided to teach whatever he had learned in his whole life to his apprentice. However, this apprentice was so arrogant that he despised his master even though he had learnt only a little bit of medical knowledge. Heart-broken, the old man let the apprentice leave to start his own business. But he also warned the young man that a kind of herb called "leafless grass" should be used cautiously because its stems and roots had different uses—its stems were used to induce perspiration while its roots could stop perspiration. Once misused, this herb would be fatal. However, the apprentice didn't pay much attention to the master's warning.

Since then, the apprentice left the master and started his own business. However, before long, one of the patients died because the apprentice misused this "rootless grass". Then the family of the deceased patient sued him for murder. After interrogation, the county magistrate found that the patient with abnormal sweating needed to be treated with roots of "leafless grass". However, the apprentice used the stems of the grass by mistake, which caused the death of the patient. Therefore, the apprentice was sentenced to prison for three years due to his negligence.

In prison, he gradually understood that the Traditional Chinese Medicine was too profound to master. He also regretted for what he had done. Therefore, he went to repent in front of his master after being released from prison. Seeing that the apprentice had changed, the master let him stay and continued to teach him medical knowledge. From then on, the apprentice was very careful when he used the "leafless grass". Since this kind of grass had got him into big trouble, he called it "Ma Fan Cao" (which literally means "troublesome grass") and later changed its name to "Ma Huang" (which literally means "troublesome yellow") because its root was yellow.

Although this is only a folklore story, it also shows that doctors cannot make even the smallest mistake when prescribing medicines to the patients. If they prescribed the wrong medicines, this would cause serious consequences. Therefore, medical work is both serious and sacred, and doctors need to treat every patient with both patience and carefulness.

蒲公英

Pugongying / Mongolian Dandelion Herb / Herba Taraxaci

知识模块

来源： 菊科（Compositae）植物蒲公英 *Taraxacum mongolicum* Hand.-Mazz.、碱地蒲公英 *T. sinicum* Kitam. 及同属多种植物的干燥带根全草。

产地： 全国大部分地区均有产地。

本草始载： 始载于唐代《新修本草》。

功效： 清热解毒，消痈散结，清利湿热。

主治： 治疗疮痈肿毒、湿热黄疸及热淋等。

Basic knowledge

Origin: The whole plant including root of *Taraxacum mongolicum* Hand.-Mazz., *T. borealisinense* Kitam. and some other species belongs to the same genus of family Compositae.

Location: Pugongying is mainly produced in most parts of China.

First recorded in: *Xin Xiu Ben Cao* (*Newly Revised Materia Medica*) of the Eastern Han Dynasty.

Efficacy: Clearing heat and removing toxicity, resolving carbuncle and stagnation, eliminating dampness and heat.

Indications: Sores and abscess, jaundice due to damp-heat, heat stranguria.

蒲公英这种常见的小草既是传统中药，又是常见的野菜，可以食用，已被收载于《既是食品又是药品的物品名单》中。它的食用价值、医药价值和营养价值在《本草纲目》等历代医药典籍中都得到了极高的评价和肯定。蒲公英不仅营养丰富，而且具有多种功效。比如，可以去火消炎、利尿散结及改善乳腺健康及改善皮肤状态等。生活中可以食用其嫩叶，可以生吃、凉拌和做馅等；用蒲公英泡茶既方便又能起到保健作用。蒲公英虽好，但是容易过敏的人、慢性肠炎患者和低血压的人要慎用蒲公英。

Related information

Pugongying, a very common weed, is not only a Chinese herbal medicine, but also a common wild vegetable that can be eaten. It has been included in List of Items That Are both Food and Medicine. Its edible value, medical value and nutritional value have been highly appraised and confirmed in the *Compendium of Materia Medica* and many other ancient medical books. It is not only nutritious, but also has a variety of effects. For example, it can clear heat and relieve

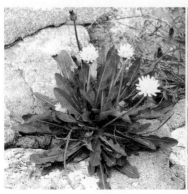 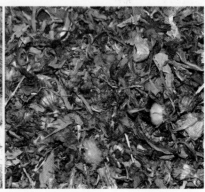

inflammation, promote diuresis and resolve stagnation, improve breast health, and improve skin condition, etc. In daily life, its tender leaves can be eaten raw, or made into salad or stuffing; Pugongying tea is also a healthy drink for people. However, those people with allergy, chronic enteritis and hypotension had better not take it.

故事模块

古时候，有一大户人家的小姐忽然得了乳疮（急性乳腺炎），但是迫于封建礼教，她不敢向郎中求医（当时只有男性郎中），后来被母亲发现了。母亲误会女儿做了越轨之事并对她破口大骂，小姐又羞又气，于是心一横就来到江边投江自尽。幸好她被一位姓蒲的老渔翁和他女儿救起。问其缘由，小姐就把患乳疮的事告诉了他们。第二天，渔家姑娘按老渔翁的指点，从山上挖回一种长着锯齿状长叶和白绒球的野草，熬成药汤给小姐喝。没过几天，小姐的病就好了。小姐的父母听说了此事，知道冤屈了女儿，来到渔船上接女儿回家。老渔翁让小姐把剩下的草药带着，如果再犯病时就煎水服用。后来，为了纪念渔家父女，因为只知老渔翁姓蒲，尊称蒲公，姑娘叫英子，就给这种药取名"蒲公英"。

Story

In ancient times, a young lady from a wealthy family suddenly got acute mastitis, but due to feudal ethics, she dared not see a doctor (because there were only male doctors during that time). After knowing this, her mother misunderstood her and blamed her for having an affair with some man. Ashamed and angry, the young lady went to the river and threw herself into the water. Luckily, she was rescued by an old fisherman surnamed Pu and his daughter. The young lady told them about her disease. The next day, with the instructions of her father, the fishergirl went to mountains and came back with a kind of herb that had long serrated leaves and white blowballs. She made a soup with this herb for the young lady. In a few days, the young lady recovered. After hearing about this, her parents knew that they had wronged their daughter and finally took the young lady home from the fishing boat. The old fisherman asked the young lady to bring the rest of the herb with her, and told her that if she got the same problem again, she would drink the soup with this herb. Later, in memory of the old fisherman and his daughter, she named this medicinal herb "Pu Gong Ying" because "Pu" was the surname of the old fisherman, "Gong" was a respectful title for the elderly men in ancient China, and "Ying" was the given name of the fishergirl.

薄荷
Bohe / Peppermint / Herba Menthae

来源：唇形科（Labiatae）植物薄荷 *Mentha haplocalyx* Briq. 的干燥地上部分。

产地：主产于江苏太仓，浙江、湖南、河南等地亦产。

本草始载：始载于唐代《新修本草》。

功效：疏散风热，清利头目，利咽，透疹，疏肝行气。

主治：治疗风热表证，麻疹不透，肝郁气滞等。

Basic knowledge

Origin: The dry aerial parts of *Mentha haplocalyx* Briq. belonging to the family Labiatae.

Location: Bohe is mainly produced in Taicang of Jiangsu Province; it is also produced in Zhejiang, Hunan and Henan provinces, etc.

First recorded in: *Xin Xiu Ben Cao* (*Newly Revised Materia Medica*) of the Tang Dynasty.

Efficacy: Dispersing wind-heat, clearing the dizziness in head and improving eyesight, relieving sore throat, promoting eruption, soothing liver and promoting flow of qi.

Indications: Exterior wind-heat syndrome, measles without adequate eruption, and stagnation of liver qi.

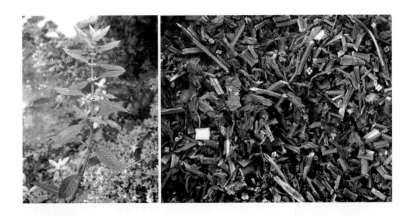

拓展模块

　　薄荷已被收载于《既是食品又是药品的物品名单》。除药用外，广泛用于食品和日化用品中。如加到糖果、糕点中以增加清凉气味，能促进食欲。但体虚多汗、脾胃虚寒和腹泻便溏者慎用。薄荷也常被加到日化用品中，如牙膏、漱口液、香水、香皂、花露水、洗发水、空气清洁剂等，能起到清洁、杀菌等作用。

Related information

Bohe has been included in List of Items That Are both Food and Medicine. Besides medicinal values, it is also widely used in food as well as household and personal care products. If added into candies and cakes, it can help to promote people's appetite because of its cool and fresh taste. However, people with excessive sweating due to deficiency of body, week spleen and stomach, and diarrhea and loose stool should be cautious when taking it. Bohe is often applied in household and personal care products, such as toothpaste, mouthwash, perfume, soap, toilet water, shampoo, air cleaner, as it has the effects of cleaning and sterilization.

故事模块

古罗马诗人奥维德在《变形记》中讲述道，水泽仙女明塔（Minthe）原本是冥界的一名侍女，但她一心梦想着自己能成为冥王哈迪斯的冥后，但不料哈迪斯却抢走了宙斯与德墨忒尔的女儿珀尔塞福涅，娶她为

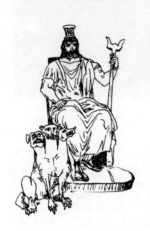

冥后，这让明塔嫉妒不已，到处传扬说自己要比珀尔塞福涅更加美丽高贵，并且一定能赢回哈迪斯，甚至扬言要将珀耳塞福涅扫地出门。愤怒的珀尔塞福涅将明塔疯狂地踩成尘土，但哈迪斯出于同情，让明塔的骨灰中长出了一种植物，并以她的名字命名为薄荷草（mentha）。早在古希腊罗马时期，薄荷就广泛应用于人们生活的各个方面，比如烹饪、入药、化妆品，甚至葬礼中。

Story

Ovid, a peot in ancient Rome, told a story in his *Metamorphosis*: Minthe, a Nymph of Cocytus river, was once a maid of the underworld, but she always dreamed of being the queen of Hades, the ruler of the underworld. However, Hades married Persephone, the daughter of Zeus and Demeter, which made Minthe extremely jealous. She told people that she was nobler and more beautiful than Persephone, and she would win Hades back. In a fury, Persephone trampled her into ashes, but out of sympathy, Hades turned her ashes into a kind of herb that bears her name "mentha" (which is called peppermint in English and Bohe in Chinese). As early as ancient Greece and Rome, Bohe was widely used in many aspects of people's life, such as cooking, medicine, cosmetics and even funeral rites.

（三）花类 / Flower

红花
Honghua / Safflower / Flos Carthami

知识模块

来源： 菊科（Compositae）植物红花 *Carthamus tinctorius* L. 的不带子房的干燥花。

产地： 主产于新疆、河南、湖南、四川等地。

本草始载： 始载于宋代《开宝本草》。

功效： 活血通经，祛瘀止痛。

主治： 治疗血瘀经闭，胸痹心痛，跌打损伤，疮痈肿痛等，可用于治疗心血管疾病。

Basic knowledge

Origin: The dry flower without ovary of *Carthamus tinctorius* L. belonging to the family Compositae.

Location: Honghua is mainly produced in Xinjiang Uygur Autonomous Region, Henan, Hunan and Sichuan provinces of China.

First recorded in: *Kai Bao Ben Cao* (*Materia Medica in Kai-Bao Reign*) of the Song Dynasty.

Efficacy: Activating blood circulation and dredging the meridian, removing blood stasis and alleviating pain.

Indications: Amenorrhea due to stasis, thoracic obstruction and cardiodynia, traumatic injuries, sores and abscess, cardiovascular disease.

红花是一种常见的保健中药，被收载于《可用于保健食品的物品名单》。红花可以泡茶泡酒，或做成药膳。此外，用红花泡脚是一种很好的养生方式。比如红花和艾叶煮水泡脚，能够活血化淤、促进血液循环，起到很好的保健作用。但并不是所有人都适合使用红花，比如孕妇、出血性疾病患者等。还有我们生活中常用到的红花油，能够治疗风湿骨痛，跌打扭伤，是一种家庭常备药。

Related information

Honghua is a common health care medicine which is included in List of Items That Can Be Used as Health Food. Honghua can be used in tea drink, soaked in wine, or cooked in food. Besides, it is a good way for people to keep fit by soaking feet in Honghua water. For example,

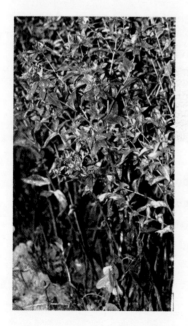

soaking feet in water boiled with Honghua and Aiye (mugwort leaves) can promote blood circulation and is a good health care method. But this method is not suitable for everyone, such as pregnant women or patients with hemorrhagic disease. Besides, the "Honghua You" (Safflower Oil) that Chinese people often use in the daily life can treat rheumatism and ostealgia, or some traumatic injuries such as sprains and bruises. It is really a kind of household medicine.

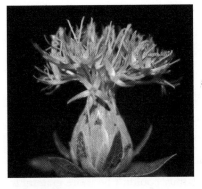
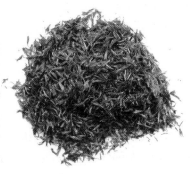

故事模块

据说古时有一位姓徐的妇女产后突然病危，家人连忙请来名医陆日严诊治，等到医生赶到病人家中时，病人几乎没有了呼吸，只有胸膛还有些微热，陆日严诊断以后考虑再三对病人家属说："此乃血闷之病，速购数十斤红花方可奏效。"没多久，红花就买来了，他便用让人大锅煮红花，等到红花水沸腾之后，把水倒入三只木桶里，再取来窗格横着放在木桶上面，然后让病人躺在窗格上用药气熏蒸。药汤冷后再倒入锅里加热，然后倒入桶中，如此反复，过了一会儿，病人僵硬的手开始活动。这样反复熏蒸半天左右，病人竟然渐渐苏醒，最终脱离了危险，全家人对这位名医都不胜感激。

Story

It is said that a woman surnamed Xu in ancient times was suddenly in danger after childbirth. Her family hurriedly sent for the famous doctor Lu Riyan. When the doctor arrived, the patient hardly breathed. Only her chest was slightly warm. After Lu Riyan's diagnosis and deep thought, he said to the family members of the patient, "This is internal hemorrhage. Buy dozens of pounds of Honghua quickly, and she might

147

be saved." After the Honghua was bought, he asked people to boil it in a large pot. After boiling, the water was poured into three wooden barrels. Then the doctor asked people to find a large piece of wood latticework and placed it on the barrels, and then he let the patient lie on the latticework so that she could be fumigated with the hot gas. When the soup was cooler, it was boiled in the pot again and then poured back into the barrels. After a while the patient's stiff hands began to move. After being fumigated for about half a day, the patient was finally out of danger, and the whole family couldn't be more grateful to this famous doctor.

金银花
Jinyinhua / Honeysuckle Bud and Flower / Flos Lonicerae

知识模块

来源：忍冬科（Caprifoliaceae）植物忍冬 *Lonicera japonica* Thunb. 的干燥花蕾。

产地：主产于山东省、河南省、河北省。

本草始载：始载于魏晋《名医别录》。

功效：清热解毒，疏散风热。

主治：治疗疮痈肿毒、风热感冒、热毒引起的痢疾。

Basic knowledge

Origin: The dry buds of *Lonicera japonica* Thunb. belonging to the family Caprifoliaceae.

Location: Jinyinhua is mainly produced in Shandong, Henan and Hebei provinces.

First recorded in: *Ming Yi Bie Lu* (*Miscellaneous Records of Famous Physicians*) of Wei-Jin Period.

Efficacy: Clearing heat and toxicity, dispelling wind-heat.

Indications: Sores and abscess, wind-heat type common cold, dysentery caused by heat-toxicity.

拓展模块

早在三千多年前，我们祖先就开始用金银花防治疾病，它在《名医别录》中被列为上品。现代生活中人们也常用它进行养生保健。金银花

149

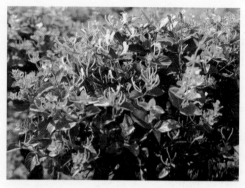 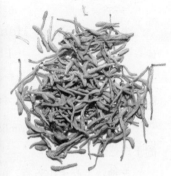

收载于《既是食品又是药品的物品名单》，由于其具有清热解毒、疏利咽喉、消暑除烦的作用，因此是岭南凉茶的主要原料之一。生活中可以喝金银花茶或金银花泡水，能够祛暑止渴，养颜美容。但是，脾胃虚寒者（如经常肚子疼、腹泻、腹部发凉、手脚发凉）不宜长期食用金银花。

＼ Related information

As early as more than 3,000 years ago, our ancestors have begun to use Jinyinhua to prevent and cure diseases. It was regarded as the top-grade medicine in *Miscellaneous Records of Famous Physicians*. In modern life, people often use it for health care. It is included in List of Items That Are both Food and Medicine. It is one of the main raw materials of herbal tea in Lingnan Region of China (South of Five Ridges) because of its functions of clearing heat and toxicity, soothing throat, relieving heat and restlessness. Jinyinhua tea can also clear summer heat, quench thirst, and nourish the skin. However, people with deficient cold of spleen and stomach (with symptoms such as frequent abdominal pain, diarrhea, abdominal cold, cold hands and feet) should not take too much of it.

故事模块

宋代张邦基在《墨庄漫录》中记载道：宋徽宗年间，奸臣蔡京、高俅专权，天灾人祸不断。苏州太平山白云寺的僧人们只好挖野菜度日，有僧人从山上采回来许多漂亮鲜美的蘑菇，可是煮食之后，许多僧人中毒。一位僧人想起有人用一种叫鸳鸯草的草药来治疗毒疮，他想即使这种草药不能解蘑菇的毒，也可以试一试。于是他便采来鸳鸯草煮水给中毒的僧侣服下，结果他们都得救了。这里所说的鸳鸯草就是金银花。

相传，药王孙思邈有一天看病归来觉得口干舌燥，他碰见两姐妹正在晒药，就向她们讨杯茶喝。孙思邈一口气喝完，只觉入口甘甜，清神气爽，便问这是什么花泡的茶。两姐妹告诉他这种花初开时是银色，久了就变成金色，所以叫金银花。孙思邈领悟到它的药性，在后来不少方剂中都以此花为主药。

金银花还具有美容的功效。据清朝《御香缥缈录》一书中记载，慈禧尤其喜欢用金银花泡茶。她睡觉前敷完"蛋清"面膜，用肥皂和清水洁面后，还会再涂上一层金银花蒸馏液，以起到美容养颜的目的。

Story

Zhang Bangji in the Song Dynasty recorded in his book *Mo Zhuang Man Lu* that during the reign of Huizong in the Song Dynasty, the two evil courtiers Cai Jing and Gao Qiu seized the real power, and the whole society suffered from a series of natural and man-made disasters. Therefore, monks at Baiyun Temple in Taiping Mountain of Suzhou had to take wild herbs for a living. Some monks picked many good-looking and delicious mushrooms from the mountains, but after taking these mushrooms, many monks became food poisoned. A monk remembered that a man had cured poisonous sores with a special herb named "mandarin duck grass". He thought he could have a try to treat the poisoned monks with this herb. So he decocted this herb in water and gave the soup to the poisoned monks. The monks who drank this soup were all saved. The herb mentioned in this story is actually Jinyinhua.

Legend has it that one day Sun Simiao, the "King of Medicine", came back from a patient's home, feeling rather thirsty. When he met the two sisters drying medicine in the sun, he asked them for a cup of tea. After drinking the tea, Sun Simiao felt that it was really sweet and refreshing. He asked what the tea was made of, and the two sisters told him that the tea was made with a special flower called "Jinyinhua" (which literally means Silver-Golden Flower) because it was silver when it first bloomed, and then became golden after some time. Sun Simiao realized its values, and later used it as the main medicine in many prescriptions.

Jinyinhua also has the beauty effect. As recorded in *Imperial Incense of the Qing Dynasty*, Empress Dowager Cixi especially liked to drink tea with it. Besides, after using "egg white" facial masks and washing her face with soap and water, she would apply some distilled liquid of Jinyinhua on her face for the sake of skin care.

菊花

Juhua / Chrysanthemum Flower / Flos Chrysanthemi

知识模块

来源：为菊科（Compositae）植物菊 *Chrysanthemum morifolium* Ramat. 的干燥头状花序。

产地：主产于浙江、安徽、河南、河北、山东等地。

本草始载：始载于东汉《神农本草经》。

功效：疏散风热，平抑肝阳，清肝明目，清热解毒。

主治：治疗风热感冒，肝阳上亢，肝火旺盛，疮痈肿毒等。

Basic knowledge

Origin: The dry flower head of *Chrysanthemum morifolium* Ramat. belonging to the family Compositae.

Location: Juhua is mainly produced in Zhejiang, Anhui, Henan, Hebei, Shandong provinces, etc.

First recorded in: *Shennong's Classic of Materia Medica* of the Eastern Han Dynasty.

Efficacy: Dispersing wind-heat, subduing liver-yang, removing liver fire for improving eyesight, clearing heat and toxicity.

Indications: Wind-heat type common cold, hyperactivity of liver-yang, exuberant fire of liver, sores and abscess.

拓展模块

菊花自古以来就一直受到人们的喜爱，在中国传统文化中扮演着重要的作用。作为药用的菊花，根据产地的不同，名字也各不相同，比如安徽亳州的"亳菊"，安徽歙县的"贡菊"，浙江桐乡的"杭白菊"，河南焦作的"怀菊"等。

菊花也是一种保健食品，被收载于《既是食品又是药品的物品名单》。它有平肝明目的功效，因此常用电脑的上班族和课业压力重的学生可以喝些菊花茶，能缓解眼睛疲劳。菊花具有散风清热的功效，可有效缓解风热感冒。此外，菊花还可以与各种茶叶、山楂、枸杞子、槐花或者金银花等一起冲泡，具有不同的功效。菊花也可以用来煮粥，气味芳香，清新爽口。但菊花性偏苦寒，体虚之人不宜多喝。

Related information

Juhua / Chrysanthemum flower has been loved by Chinese people since ancient times and plays an important role in traditional Chinese culture. Different kinds of chrysanthemum for medicinal use have different names according to their places of production, such as "Bo Ju" from Bozhou of Anhui Province, "Gong Ju" from Shexian of Anhui Province, "Hangbai Ju" from Tongxiang of Zhejiang Province, and "Huai Ju" from Jiaozuo of Henan Province and so on.

Juhua is also a health care food included in List of Items That Are both Food and Medicine. It has the effects of suppressing hyperactive liver and improving the eyesight, so the office workers who often use

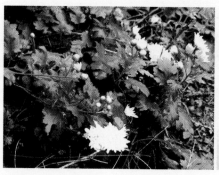
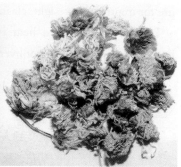

computers and students who are under pressure from their schoolwork can drink some Juhua tea to relieve eye fatigue. Chrysanthemum has the effect of dispersing wind and clearing heat, and it can effectively relieve wind heat common cold. Besides, it can also be brewed together with tea leaves, Shanzha (hawthorn fruit), Gouqizi (wolfberry fruit), Huaihua (sophora flower) or Jinyinhua (honeysuckle flower) with different effects. It can also be used to make porridge, which tastes fragrant and refreshing. But it is bitter and cold, and is not suitable for people with weak constitution.

故事模块

关于菊花的故事，在我国民间流传很多。早在两千多年前，汉代应劭在《风俗通义》里记载说河南南阳郦县有个叫甘谷的村庄，谷中水甜美，山上长着许多菊花，一股山泉从山上菊花从中流过，花瓣散落水中，使水含有菊花的清香，村里三十多户人家都饮用这泉水，一般都活到130岁，最低的也有七八十岁。

当然，饮用菊花水就能活到130岁，这只是杜撰的故事而已。但自古以来，菊花就一直受到人们的喜爱和重视。

比如《神农本草经》中记载："菊花久服能轻身延年"。汉朝的《西京杂记》记载了如何酿制菊花酒，而且当时帝宫后妃皆称之为"长寿酒"，把它当作滋补药品。三国时期，蜀国人多种菊，以苗入菜，以花入药。曹操的儿子魏文帝曹丕，有一年重阳节的时候给他的好友，也是书法家和政治家的钟繇写了一封谈论菊花的信——《九日与钟繇书》。信中写到，又到了九月九日，秋天草木凋谢，只有菊花不惧寒冷"纷然独荣"，可见它"含乾坤之纯和"，是可以让人延年益寿的好东西，因此送给他一束菊花，以供他研究"彭祖之术"，即长寿的道理（据传彭祖活了八百岁）。

东晋著名诗人陶渊明爱菊成癖，写过不少咏菊的诗句，如著名的"采菊东篱下，悠然见南山"。他也提到了服用菊花对于健康的重要性，例如他在《九日闲居》中提到"酒能祛百虑，菊解制颓龄"。由此可见，古人爱菊，不但观赏，也早就认识到菊的药用和食用价值。

Story

There are many stories about Juhua in China. As early as 2,000 years ago, Ying Shao of the Han Dynasty recorded in his book *Feng Su Tong Yi (The Study of Customs)* that there was a village named Gangu in Nanyang, Henan Province. The water in the valley was sweet, and there were many chrysanthemums growing all over the mountains. A mountain spring flowed through the chrysanthemums and their petals scattered in the water, which made the water contain the fragrance of chrysanthemum flowers. There were more than 30 families in the village, and these people all drank the spring water. They generally lived to 130 years old, and even the lowest life expectancy was seventy or eighty years.

Of course, it is just a fabricated story that drinking chrysanthemum water can help people live to 130 years old. But since ancient times, chrysanthemum has been loved and valued by people.

For example, *Shennong's Classic of Materia Medica* points out that "taking chrysanthemum for a long time will help people to keep healthy and prolong life". How to make chrysanthemum wine was recorded in *Xi Jing Za Ji (A Miscellany of the Western Capital)* of the Han Dynasty. At that time, the royal family members called it "Longevity Wine", and used it as a nourishing medicine. During the Three Kingdoms Period, people in Shu State have planted many kinds of chrysanthemums. They used its seedlings for food and flowers for medicine. Cao Cao's son Cao Pi, Emperor Wen of the Wei State, wrote a letter about chrysanthemum to his friend Zhong Yao, a calligrapher and politician. The letter was titled A Letter to Zhong Yao on the Double Ninth Festival. It was written in the letter that on September 9th, when all the plants withered in autumn, only the chrysanthemum did not fear the cold and was "blooming alone". Apparently it contained "the pure harmony of heaven and earth", and thus it was a good thing for people to prolong their lives. Therefore, he sent a bunch of chrysanthemums to Zhong Yao for him to study "Peng Zu's secret", that is, the secret of longevity (Peng Zu lived for over 800 years according to ancient legend).

Tao Yuanming, a poet of the Eastern Jin Dynasty (317−420), was crazy about chrysanthemum and wrote many poems about it, such as the most famous verse "While picking asters' neath the Eastern fence, my gaze upon the Southern mountain rests". He has realized the importance of taking chrysanthemum for health care, such as "Wine can dispel all worries, while chrysanthemum can delay my aging" in his poem Nine Days of Leisure. It can be seen from these examples that the ancients have always been fond of chrysanthemum, and have already recognized its values as an ornamental, medicinal and edible plant.

（四）果实种子类 / Fruit and Seed

大枣
Dazao / Chinese Dates / Fructus Jujubae

知识模块

来源: 鼠李科(Rhamnaceae)植物枣 *Ziziphus jujuba* Mill. 的成熟果实。

产地: 主产于河北、河南、山东、新疆等地。

本草始载: 始载于东汉《神农本草经》。

功效: 补中益气，养血安神，缓和药性。

主治: 治疗脾胃虚弱及失眠等。

Basic knowledge

Origin: The ripe fruit of *Ziziphus jujuba* Mill. belonging to the family Rhamnaceae.

Location: Dazao is mainly produced in Hebei, Henan, Shandong provinces, and Xinjiang Uygur Autonomous Region, etc.

First recorded in: *Shenong's Classic of Materia Medica* of the Eastern Han Dynasty

Efficacy: Invigorating spleen-stomach and replenishing qi, nourishing blood for tranquillization, relieving violent property of some herbs.

Indications: Spleen and stomach deficiency, insomnia.

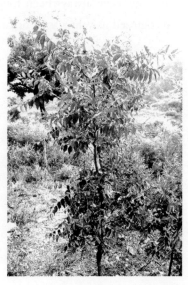

拓展模块

大枣是一味非常常见的药食两用佳品，收载于《既是食品又是药品的物品名单》。它营养丰富，能够补脾、养血、安神，常吃大枣，还能让人面色红润，达到美容养颜的目的。可以用来泡茶、煮粥、炖汤等。但是大枣虽好，却不可过量食用，特别是肠胃不好的人一定不能多吃，否则会引起腹胀。此外，大枣糖分丰富，不适合糖尿病患者。

Related information

Dazao, with a dual usage of food and medicine, is included in List of Items That Are both Food and Medicine. Rich in nutrients, it can tonify the spleen, nourish blood, and tranquilize the mind. Eating Dazao regularly can also help people have a ruddy complexion, which helps to nourish your beauty. It can be used to make tea, porridge, stew and so on. However, although it has a lot of benefits for people, it cannot be eaten excessively, especially for those with a poor stomach; otherwise they will get abdominal distension. In addition, it is rich in sugar and is not suitable for people with diabetics.

故事模块

一提到大枣，大家想到的就是它的补血功能，其实大枣的功效可不止补血。

宋代医学家陈自明整理编辑了宋代以前的妇产科著作，并撰写了一本《妇人良方》，书里记载了这样一个病例，有一位妇人经常在白天悲哭，可是又说不出原因，试过多种方法都没有什么效果。有位郎中诊断此症为"脏躁"，告诉她只需要服用大枣汤，悲戚的情绪自然就会停止，果然这位妇人在服用大枣汤后很快就痊愈了。

张仲景在《金匮要略》中道："妇人脏躁，喜悲伤欲哭，像如神灵所作（像鬼神附体一般），数欠伸（总打呵欠），甘麦大枣汤主之。用甘缓之品，可以缓其情志剧烈波动。"前文提到的妇人所用的大枣汤即张仲景的甘麦大枣汤，因此能对那位妇人起到立竿见影的效果。

Story

When it comes to Dazao, it is considered as a blood tonic. In fact, it has many other effects besides nourishing the blood.

Chen Ziming, a medical expert of the Song Dynasty, edited the works of gynecology and obstetrics before Song Dynasty, and compiled a book titled *Fu Ren Liang Fang* (*A Complete Book of Effective Prescription for Women*). A case was recorded in this book. A woman often cried sadly during the day and couldn't tell why. She tried many methods but all in vain. One doctor diagnosed that her problem was "Zang Zao" (which is similar to hysteria), and what she needed was Dazao Soup. Luckily, she recovered soon after taking Dazao Soup.

Zhang Zhongjing mentioned in his famous classic *Jingui Yaolue* (*Synopsis of Golden Chamber*), "When a women gets Zang Zao, she will feel depressed and always cry as if she was haunted by the spirits. And

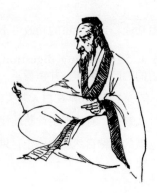

she will also yawn a lot. Ganmai Dazao Soup could be used to treat her because Gancao (liquorice root), Xiaomai (wheat) and Dazao could alleviate the grief and restlessness." The Dazao Soup taken by the above-mentioned woman was exactly the Ganmai Dazao Soup introduced by Zhang Zhongjing, so it had the immediate effect on the patient.

山楂

Shanzha / Hawthorn Fruit / Fructus Crataegi

知识模块

来源： 蔷薇科（Rosaceae）多年生落叶灌木或小乔木山楂 *Crataegus pinnatifida* Bge. 和山里红 *C. pinnatifida* Bge. var. *major* N. E. Br. 的干燥成熟果实。

产地： 主产于山东、河北、河南、辽宁等地。

本草始载： 始载于唐代《新修本草》。

功效： 消食健胃，行气散瘀。

主治： 治疗饮食积滞，瘀血阻滞。

Basic knowledge

Origin: The dry ripe fruit of perennial deciduous shrubs or small arbor plant *Crataegus pinnatifida* Bge. and *C. pinnatifida* Bge. var. *major* N. E. Br. belonging to the family Rosaceae.

Location: Shanzha is mainly produced in Shandong, Hebei, Henan, and Liaoning provinces, etc.

First recorded in: *Xin Xiu Ben Cao* (*Newly Revised Materia Medica*) of the Tang dynasty.

Efficacy: Relieving food stagnation and improving digestion, regulating qi and resolving stasis.

Indications: Food stagnation and blood stasis.

拓展模块

山楂是一味药食两用品种,收载于《既是食品又是药品的物品名单》。有一种长得和山楂极为相似的水果名叫山里红,又称红果,是山楂的变种,果实个大而面,酸度略小,多为食用,像大家熟知的京津地区的名小吃冰糖葫芦,就是用山里红裹上冰糖熬制好的糖浆做成的。而山楂比山里红个头小,更酸一些,一般药用较多,为消食滞的常用药。此外,山楂对高血压、高血脂、冠心病等心血管疾病也有一定疗效,可以作保健品使用。但是由于山楂含有较多的维生素 C 和枸橼酸,所以胃酸过多或胃肠溃疡的病人不宜多食。

Related information

Shanzha / hawthorn fruit can be used as both medicine and food, and it is included in List of Items That Are both Food and Medicine. There is a fruit which looks like Shanzha very much. Its name is Shanlihong (the fruit of a plant whose Latin name is Crataegus pinnatifida Bge. var. major N. E. Brown.), also known as Hongguo (which literally means red fruit), and it is a variety of Shanzha. Shanlihong is bigger and softer, and is often used as food. Like the snack named "tanghulu", or "sugar-coated haws on a stick" which is popular in Beijing and Tianjin. It is made of Shanlihong wrapped in sugar syrup. On the other hand, Shanzha is smaller and sourer than Shanlihong. It is commonly used for medicinal purposes, and is commonly used for eliminating food stagnation. In addition, Shanzha has certain effect on cardiovascular diseases such as hypertension, hyperlipidemia, coronary heart disease, and can also be used as a health care product. However, because Shanzha contains much vitamin C and citric acid, patients with hyperacidity or gastrointestinal ulcer should not eat too much of it.

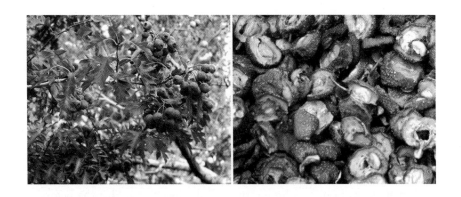

故事模块

据说南宋绍熙年间，宋光宗最宠爱的贵妃突然生病了，整日没有胃口不思饮食，因而变得面黄肌瘦，失去了往日的美丽。这可把宋光宗急坏了，他命御医们全力为这位贵妃诊治，但是御医们用了许多贵重药品，都不见效。于是，宋光宗只好贴出告示，悬赏招纳天下良医，如若治好贵妃的病，必有重赏。一位江湖郎中看到了告示，便揭榜进宫自告奋勇为贵妃治病。他为贵妃诊脉后说："治此病并不难，只要将山楂和红糖煎熬，每次饭前吃五至十枚，半月后病准会好。"贵妃按此法服用后，果然不久便病愈了。后来，这酸脆香甜的蘸糖山楂传入了民间，就慢慢演变成了深受大家喜爱的冰糖葫芦了。

Story

It is said that during the Shaoxi reign of the Southern Song Dynasty, the emperor's favorite imperial concubine was sick. She had no appetite, and didn't want to eat anything. Therefore, she became skinny with a yellow complexion, and lost her beauty. The anxious emperor ordered the royal doctors to try every means to treat her. The doctors applied many valuable medicines, but none of them were effective. Therefore, the emperor put up a notice to look for a skilled doctor from the whole country. If someone could cure the imperial concubine, he would get a lot of money as reward. A doctor saw the notice and wanted to have a try. He took the emperor's notice, went into the palace. After checking the concubine's pulse, he said, "It's not difficult to cure the disease. Boil Shanzha fruits in melted brown sugar. Take five to ten Shanzha before each meal. In half a month, she'll be all right." After taking this method, the concubine gradually recovered. Later, this sour and sweet sugared Shanzha was taken outside the royal family, and then evolved into the "sugar-coated haws on a stick" which was very popular among the common public.

五味子
Wuweizi / Chinese Magnoliavine Fruit /
Fructus Schisandrae Chinensis

知识模块

来源：木兰科（Magnoliaceae）植物五味子 *Schisandra chinensis* (Turcz.) Baill. 或华中五味子 *S. sphenanthera* Rehd. et Wils. 的成熟果实。前者习称"北五味子"，后者习称"南五味子"。

产地：北五味子主产于东北，南五味子主产于西南及长江流域以南各地。

本草始载：始载于东汉《神农本草经》。

功效：收敛固涩，益气滋肾，生津止渴，宁心安神。

主治：治疗久泻不止，久咳虚喘，遗精，自汗盗汗，心神不宁等。

Basic knowledge

Origin: The ripe fruit of either *Schisandra chinensis* (Turcz.) Baill. or *S. sphenanthera* Rehd. et Wils. belonging to the family Magnoliaceae. The former is called "Bei (North) Wuweizi" while the latter is called "Nan (South) Wuweizi".

Location: Bei Wuweizi is mainly produced in Northeast of China, while Nan Wuweizi is mainly produced in Southwest of China and the areas South of the Yangzi River.

First recorded in: *Shennong's Classic of Materia Medica* of the Eastern Han Dynasty.

Efficacy: Astringent, benefiting qi and nourishing kidney, promoting the production of body fluid to relieve thirst, calming heart and inducing tranquilization.

Indications: Chronic diarrhea, chronic cough and panting, seminal emission, spontaneous sweating and night sweating, restlessness.

╲拓展模块

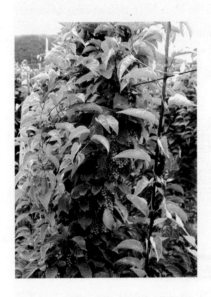

五味子是一味可以强身健体的中药，被收载于《可用于保健食品的物品名单》，一直受到养生人士的喜爱。泡水喝是五味子最为常见的保健用法，能够治疗咳嗽、痰多、失眠、潮热虚汗的毛病，还能降血压，对于肝细胞也有很好的保护作用。每天可以搭配枸杞子泡水喝1~2次，不过毕竟"是药三分毒"，五味子也有一些副作用，比如恶心、呕吐、过敏、发热、困倦乏力、反酸等，因此不能一次性服用太多的量，每次可以根据自己的需求放5至10粒即可。

╲Related information

Wuweizi is a Chinese herbal medicine which can help people to keep fit. Included in List of Items That Can Be Used as Health Food, it has always been popular among health-conscious people. It is a very common health care method to drink water with Wuweizi as it can treat cough, phlegm, insomnia, hot flashes and abnormal sweating due

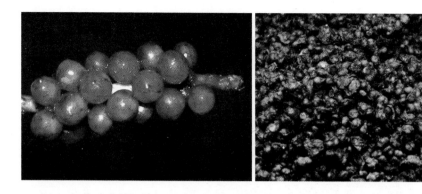

to general debility. It can also help lower high blood pressure, and is good for liver cells. People can drink water soaked with Wuweizi and Gouqizi (wolfberry fruit) 1～2 times a day. However, just like the Chinese saying that "all kinds of medicines are poisonous to various extents", Wuweizi also has some side effects, such as nausea, vomiting, allergy, fever, sleepiness, fatigue, sour regurgitation and so on. Therefore, people cannot take too much of it at one time. You can use 5 to 10 pills each time according to your own needs.

＼故事模块

　　关于五味子有一个民间故事。相传很久以前，长白山下的村庄里有一个叫苦娃的青年，他自幼父母双亡，靠给一个姓刁的员外做苦工度日。刁员外经常虐待苦娃，几年下来，苦娃得了一身的病，骨瘦如柴。一天，刁员外看苦娃的病越来越重，就派家丁将苦娃扔在树林里。气息奄奄的苦娃无意间发现了一种野果子，他饿得难以忍受，便随手摘了一串野果塞进嘴里，只觉得这种野果甘、酸、辛、苦、咸五味俱全，非常爽口。苦娃吃完之后感到精神焕发，他的病竟然被这些野果子治好了。因为这种果子有5种味道，苦娃就给它取名"五味子"。

　　这个故事只是民间传说，但事实上这种药名叫五味子，确实和它有

"酸、甜、苦、辣、咸"五种味道有关系。它的名称由来和宋朝名医苏颂有关，苏颂曾经这样形容过五味子："五味皮肉甘酸，核中辛苦，都有咸味，此则五味具也。"

Story

There is a folk story about Wuweizi. Legend has it that long ago, in the village under Changbai Mountain, there was a young man called Ku Wa (which literally means "miserable boy"). His parents died at an early age, and he had to do slave labor for a land lord surnamed Diao. Having been abused for years, Ku Wa was sick and skinny. One day, seeing that Ku Wa was incurable, Diao told his servants to leave Ku Wa in the woods. The dying young man accidentally spotted a kind of wild fruit, and he was so hungry that he picked a bunch of these wild fruits and swallowed them. He just felt the fruit was refreshing with five tastes including sweet, sour, pungent, bitter and salty. After he finished eating, he felt refreshed and his illness was cured by these wild fruits. Because this fruit had five different tastes, Ku Wa named it "Wu Wei Zi" which literally means seeds with five tastes.

Although this is only a folklore story, the name of this medicine is indeed related to its five tastes. Its name has something to do with Su Song, a famous doctor in the Song Dynasty. Su Song once described that Wuweizi had "five tastes including sweet and sour tastes in pericarp and flesh, pungent taste in kernel, and salty taste in all the parts".

连翘

Lianqiao / Weeping Forsythia Capsule / Fructus Forsythiae

知识模块

来源：木犀科（Oleaceae）植物连翘 *Forsythia suspensa* (Thunb.) Vahl 的干燥果实。主产于山西、河南、陕西等地。

产地：主产于山西、河南、陕西等地。

本草始载：始载于东汉《神农本草经》。

功效：清热解毒，消肿散结，疏散风热。

主治：治疗疮痈肿毒，风热感冒。

Basic knowledge

Origin: The dry fruit of *Forsythia suspensa* (Thunb.) Vahl belonging to the family Oleaceae.

Location: Lianqiao is mainly produced in Shanxi, Henan, and Shaanxi provinces.

First recorded in: *Shennong's Classic of Materia Medica* of the Eastern Han Dynasty

Efficacy: Clearing heat and removing toxicity, relieving swelling and dissipating nodulation, dispersing wind-heat.

Indications: Sores and abscess, wind-heat type common cold.

拓展模块

连翘是一种固沙和抗风沙植物，可有效防止水土流失，对保护黄土高原脆弱的生态环境有不可替代的作用。此外，连翘花于早春盛开，非常美丽，现在很多地方也将连翘作为园林绿化树种，用来美化环境。

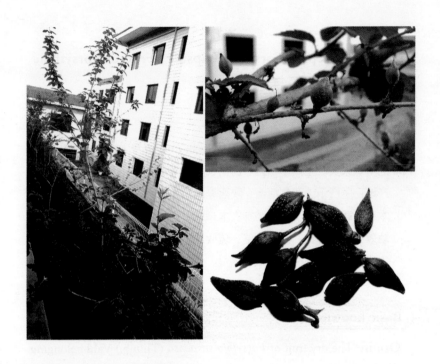

Related information

Lianqiao is a sand-fixing and sand-resisting plant which can effectively prevent soil erosion and plays an irreplaceable role in protecting the fragile ecological environment of the Loess Plateau. In addition, its beautiful flowers bloom in early spring, and therefore many Lianqiao trees are planted in many places to beautify the environment.

故事模块

岐伯是远古时代最著名的医学家,中医学奠基之作《黄帝内经》的主要内容就是以黄帝与岐伯间问答的形式写成的。中医也被称为"岐黄之术",岐就是指岐伯,黄就是指黄帝。

在河南新密市的岐伯山上有一座岐伯墓，墓东侧有一个地方叫大臣沟，沟里种着很多连翘。关于连翘，还流传着一个与岐伯有关的故事。

相传，五千年前岐伯在这里采药、种药，他有个孙女叫连翘。一天岐伯和连翘上山采药时，岐伯亲自尝验一种草药，可是却不幸中毒，口吐白沫，不省人事。连翘看爷爷生命垂危，一直哭喊着："救命！救命！"可是呼喊了好久也无人应答，心急之下她突然想到山中长着许多药材，说不定身边的这种植物也能治病救人，便急中生智顺手捋了一把植物的绿叶，揉碎后塞进爷爷的嘴里。片刻之后，岐伯慢慢苏醒过来，等到他把绿叶咽下后，竟然慢慢地恢复了。

之后岐伯就开始研究起这种植物来，经过多次试验，他发现这绿叶有较好的清热解毒作用，便把这植物收入他的中药名录，以孙女的名字为它命名为连翘，又在他居住的大臣沟里栽种了许多连翘以造福百姓。

当然这只是个民间故事，事实上连翘的入药部位是它的果实，口服也不会有解毒的功效，而是常用于治疗风热感冒等症，比如人们感冒时常吃的中成药"银翘解毒片"就含有金银花、连翘等清热解毒的中药。

Story

Qi Bo is one of the most famous doctors in ancient China. *Huang Di Nei Jing* (*Yellow Emperor's Canon of Medicine*), the classic which laid the foundation for TCM, was written in the form of questions and answers between Huang Di (Yellow Emperor) and Qi Bo. TCM is also known as "Qi Huang". "Qi" refers to Qi Bo, and "Huang" refers to Huang Di.

On Qi Bo Mountain in Xinmi City of Henan Province, there is a Qi Bo tomb. On the east side of the tomb, there is a place called Dachen Ditch, where a lot of Lianqiao bushes are planted. There is a story of Liangqiao and Qi Bo.

According to legend, five thousand years ago, Qi Bo was collecting and planting medical herbs in this place with his granddaughter named Lian Qiao. One day when Qi Bo and Lian Qiao went up to the mountain to collect medicinal herbs, Qi Bo tasted a kind of herb, but unfortunately he got poisoned, foaming at the mouth, and then became unconscious. Seeing that her Grandpa was in danger, Lian Qiao cried, "Help! Help!" But there was no one around. In a hurry, she noticed a plant near her, and thought there were many medicinal herbs in the mountain, and it was possible this plant also had curative effects. Therefore, she crumbed a handful of green leaves of this plant, and put them into Grandpa's mouth. After a moment, Qi Bo slowly came to himself. After he had swallowed the green leaves, he slowly recovered.

Then Qibo began to study these green leaves. After many experiments, he found that these green leaves had heat-clearing and detoxifying effects. Therefore, he put this plant into his list of herbal medicines, and named it "Lianqiao" after his granddaughter, and planted many of this plant in the ditch where he lived in order to benefit the common people.

Of course, this is only a folk story. In fact, the medicinal part of Lianqiao is its fruit. Taking its leaves orally cannot cure poisoning as

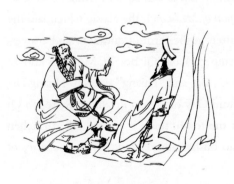

described in the story. Actually, it is often used to treat wind-heat type cold. For example, the Chinese patent medicine Yinqiao Jiedu Tablet, which people often take when they catch cold, contains Jinyinhua, Lianqiao and other medicines.

陈皮

Chenpi / Dried Tangerine Peel / Pericarpium Citri Reticulatae

知识模块

来源：芸香科（Rutaceae）植物橘 *Citrus reticulata* Blanco 及栽培变种的干燥成熟果皮。

产地：主产于广东、福建、四川、江苏、浙江、江西、湖南、云南、贵州等地。

本草始载：始载于东汉《神农本草经》。

功效：理气健脾，燥湿化痰。

主治：治疗胸脘胀满，吐泻，咳嗽痰多。

Basic knowledge

Origin: The dry ripe pericarp of *Citrus reticulata* Blanco and its cultivar belonging to the family Rutaceae.

Location: Chenpi is mainly produced in Guangdong, Fujian, Sichuan, Jiangsu, Zhejiang, Jiangxi, Hunan, Yunnan, Guizhou provinces, etc.

First recorded in: *Shennong's Classic of Materia Medica* of the Eastern Han Dynasty.

Efficacy: Promoting flow of qi, invigorating spleen, drying dampness and resolving phlegm.

Indications: Chest fullness, vomiting, diarrhea, cough, and phlegm.

拓展模块

陈皮讲究的就是一个"陈"字。越陈越好！药用的陈皮最少需要陈制一年才能使用，广东新会陈皮甚至要求陈制三年以上。中医认为新鲜的橘皮性烈，含有较多挥发油，会对消化道产生刺激，可能诱发胃肠道疾病，所以需要陈制后才能成为理气燥湿化痰的中药。2011年首届新会陈皮文化节上，1929年产的广东新会陈皮竟然以每公斤110万元的价格成功拍出天价。

陈皮的原料橘皮被载入《既是食品又是药品名单》。陈皮一直以来也是人们喜爱的养生食材，有镇咳祛痰、提高食欲及降血压等功效，因此有"一两陈皮一两金"的说法。陈皮最简单的用法就是陈皮切丝，沸水冲泡，可以健脾和胃，行气化痰；再比如陈皮和姜一起泡水喝可以缓解感冒症状；陈皮山楂红枣茶有驱寒暖胃的作用。此外，陈皮也可用来煮粥炖汤。

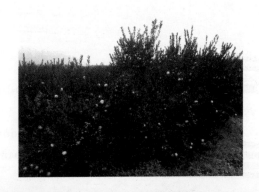

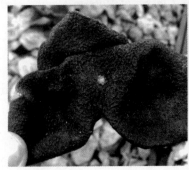
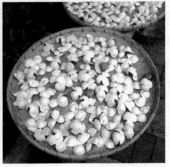

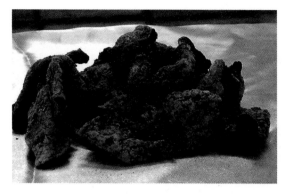

价值 110 万 / 公斤的陈皮

Related information

The Chinese name of dried tangerine peel is "Chenpi", and "Chen" means "old" or "aged" in Chinese. Actually, the older the Chenpi is, the better effects it will have. Chenpi should be aged for at least one year, and the "Xinhui Chenpi" produced in Xinhui of Guangdong Province must be aged for over three years. According to Chinese medicine theory, the fresh tangerine peel contains much volatile oil which can be irritating to the digestive tract and thus might induce gastrointestinal diseases. Therefore, it needs to be aged before it can become a Chinese medicine with the effects of regulating qi, drying dampness and resolving phlegm. At the first Xinhui Chenpi Culture Festival in 2011, the Chenpi produced in 1929 was sold at the price of 1.1 million *Yuan* per kilogram.

The tangerine peel, the raw material of Chenpi, is included in List of Items That Are both Food and Medicine. Chenpi has always been a popular health food, with antitussive and expectorant effects, and also the effects of improving appetite and lowering blood pressure. There is a saying that one liang of Chenpi is worth one liang of gold (1 liang is equal to 50 grams). The simplest method to use Chenpi is to cut it into fine shreds and brew them with boiling water. This may invigorate the spleen and stomach, activate qi, and relieve phlegm; besides, drinking water soaked with Chenpi and ginger can alleviate cold; Chenpi-Shanzha-Dazao tea (soak Chenpi, hawthorn fruit and Chinese dates in boiling water) has the function of dispelling cold and warming the stomach. In addition, Chenpi can also be used in porridge or soup.

故事模块

相传宋朝天圣元年，范仲淹在东台任盐仓监官，当时他的母亲体弱多病，但又怕苦，不愿服用汤药。为此，范仲淹一筹莫展，忧心忡忡，四处求医寻找治病的良方。有一天，当地的一位名医给了范仲淹一味良方：用糯米配以中药，制成药酒饮用。于是，范仲淹立刻找来中药请人调制药酒，范仲淹的母亲饮用后果然身体逐渐康复起来。

第二年冬天接连下雪，天气寒冷，许多修筑堤坝的工人都生病了，范仲淹就令人配制这种药酒给工人服用，工人们饮用后不久也都病愈了。这种药酒就是以糯米为原料，配以陈皮等十六种药物制成。

Story

Legend has it that in the first year of Tiansheng years of the Song Dynasty, Fan Zhongyan served as the salt warehouse inspector in Dongtai. At that time, his mother was sick but refused to take the bitter soup medicine. Therefore, Fan Zhongyan was helpless and worried, seeking medical advice everywhere to find a cure. One day, a famous local doctor gave Fan Zhongyan a good prescription, i.e. to make a kind of medicinal wine with glutinous rice and some Chinese herbal medicines. Therefore, Fan Zhongyan immediately asked people to buy the necessary medicines and make this medicinal wine. His mother gradually recovered after drinking it.

The next winter it was very cold as it snowed for many days without stopping, and many workers who built the dam got sick. Fan Zhongyan asked people to prepare this kind of medicinal wine for the workers. They also recovered soon after drinking the wine. This kind of medicinal wine is made from glutinous rice and sixteen kinds of drugs including Chenpi as one of the main ingredients.

枸杞子

Gouqizi / Wolfberry Fruit / Fructus Lycii

知识模块

来源： 茄科（Solanaceae）植物宁夏枸杞 *Lycium barbarum* L. 的干燥成熟果实。

产地： 主产于宁夏、甘肃、青海、新疆、内蒙古及河北等地。

本草始载： 始载于东汉《神农本草经》。

功效： 补肝肾，益精血，明目。

主治： 治疗肝肾阴虚导致的腰膝酸软、眩晕耳鸣、血虚萎黄、目昏不明。

Basic knowledge

Origin: The dry ripe fruit of *Lycium barbarum* L. belonging to the family Solanaceae.

Location: Gouqizi is mainly produced in Ningxia Hui Autonomous Region, Gansu Province, Qinghai Province, Xinjiang Uygur Autonomous Region, Inner Mongolia Autonomous Region, and Hebei Province, etc.

First recorded in: *Shenong's Classic of Materia Medica* of the Eastern Han Dynasty.

Efficacy: Tonifying liver and kidney, benefiting essence and blood, improving eyesight.

Indications: Soreness and limpness of lumbar and knees due to liver and kidney deficiency, dizziness and tinnitus, blood deficiency, blurred vision.

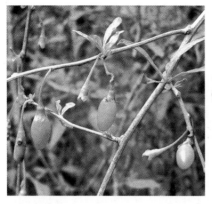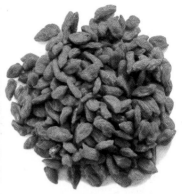

拓展模块

　　枸杞子是一味我国民间常用的药食两用佳品，收载于原卫生部颁布的《既是食品又是药品的物品名单》。枸杞子中含有丰富的氨基酸、维生素、多糖等特殊营养成分，具有非常好的保健功效，常用于药膳、食疗的保健中，比如可以泡水、煮粥、炖汤等。此外，目前流行的黑枸杞和枸杞可不是一回事哦！它和枸杞是同属但不同种的植物，黑枸杞富含花青素，具有很好的抗疲劳和抗衰老作用，同样是一个很不错的保健品。

Related information

　　Gouqizi is both food and medicine commonly used by Chinese people. It has been included in List of Items That Are both Food and Medicine issued by Ministry of Health. It contains abundant amino acids, vitamins, polysaccharides and other special nutrients. It has very good health effects and is often used in medicinal diet and dietary therapy. For example, it can be used in various health care tea, porridge and soup. In addition, the popular Heigouqi (Lycium Ruthenicum fruit) is different from Gouqizi as they are different species even though they both belong to the genus Lycium. However, Heigouqi is also a good health care product since it is rich in anthocyanins and has a good anti-fatigue and anti-aging effect.

故事模块

我国宋代医家王怀隐等人编写的《太平圣惠方》一书中讲述了一则有关枸杞子的故事。据说有一个人出使西河，在路上碰到一名女子，看上去也就十五六岁的样子，却正在打一个年约八、九十岁的老人。使者深感奇怪，便问女子："此老人是何人？"女子说："我曾孙。打之何怪？此有良药不肯服食，致使年老不能行步，所以决罚。"使者又问那女子年龄，女子说她已经372岁了。使者又问她良药有几种，女子回答说，药只有一种，但却有五个名字，春名天精，夏名枸杞，秋名地骨，冬名仙杖，也叫王母杖。经常服用能够延年益寿。

故事中的女子竟然活到300多岁，这显然是虚构出来的传奇故事，但却反映出古人早已知悉枸杞健身延年的功效。比如古代许多文人墨客，如唐代诗人陆龟蒙、刘禹锡，宋代诗人苏东坡、陆游等经常服用枸杞子进行养生，还写下了许多有关枸杞的诗句。如刘禹锡就描述枸杞为"上品功能甘露味，还知一勺可延龄"，就是说枸杞不仅味道甘甜，还可延年益寿。此外，南北朝的葛洪和陶弘景以及唐代的孙思邈等都是医林寿星，据说他们有常食枸杞的习惯。民间也流传有"要想眼睛亮，常喝枸杞汤"的俗语。因此，亲爱的读者们，你们也想尝试一下枸杞的神奇功效吗？

Story

Wang Huaiyin, a medical expert in the Song Dynasty, wrote a book called *Tai Ping Sheng Hui Fang* (*Taiping Holy Prescriptions for Universal Relief*). In this book, there is a story about Gouqizi. It is said that a man was on a mission to a place called Xihe. He came across a woman on the way. She looked only fifteen or sixteen years old, but was beating an old man who looked about eighty or ninety years old. The messenger was so surprised that he asked the woman, "Who is this old man?" The woman said, "He is my great-grandson. What's wrong with it? He refused to take the good medicine, and thus became too old to walk. That's why I decided to punish him." The messenger asked about the woman's age. The woman answered she was already 372 years old. The messenger then asked her how many kinds of good medicines she had taken. The woman answered that there was only one kind of medicine, but with five names in different seasons: Tianjing in spring, Gouqi in summer, Digu in autumn, and Xianzhang (which literally means the immortal's walking stick) in winter, also known as the Wangmuzhang (which literally means Queen Mother's walking stick). If regularly used, it can prolong life.

It is obviously a fictional story that the women lived to more than 300 years old, but the story also shows that the ancients have long known the efficacy of Gouqizi. For example, many ancient men of letters, such as Lu Guimeng and Liu Yuxi of the Tang Dynasty, Su Dongpo and Lu You of the Song Dynasty, often took Gouqizi for health care, and wrote many poems about it. For example, Liu Yuxi said Gouqizi was not only tasty as sweet dew, but also good to prolong life expectancy. In addition, Ge Hong and Tao Hongjing of the Northern and Southern Dynasties and Sun Simiao of the Tang Dynasty were all medical experts who enjoyed longevity. They were said to have a habit of taking Gouqizi. There is also a popular saying that if you want to have bright eyes, you had better often drink Gouqizi water. So my dear readers, do you want to have a try of Gouqizi?

砂仁

Sharen / Villous Amomum Fruit / Fructus Amomi Villosi

来源：为姜科（Zingiberaceae）多年生草本植物阳春砂 *Amomum villosum* Lour.、绿壳砂 *A. villosum* Lour. var. *xanthioides* T. L. Wu et Senjen 或海南砂 *A. longiligulare* T. L. Wu 的干燥成熟果实。

产地：主产于广东、广西、云南、海南及闽南地区。

本草始载：始载于唐代《本草拾遗》。

功效：化湿开胃，温中止泻，行气安胎。

主治：湿浊中阻，脾胃虚寒，泄泻呕吐，胎动不安等症。

Basic knowledge

Origin: The dry ripe fruit or of *Amomum villosum* Lour., *A. villosum* Lour. var. *xanthioides* T. L. Wu et Senje, or *A. longiligulare* T. L. Wu belonging to the family Zingiberaceae.

Location: Sharen is mainly produced in Guangdong Province, Guangxi Zhuang Autonomous Region, Yunnan Province, Hainan Province and southern part of Fujian Province.

First recorded in: *Ben Cao Shi Yi (A Supplement to Materia Medica)* of the Tang Dynasty.

Efficacy: Resolving dampness, stimulating appetite, harmonizing middle energizer, stopping diarrhea, activating qi and preventing miscarriage.

Indications: The syndrome of obstruction of dampness in middle energizer, deficiency-cold of spleen and stomach, diarrhea, vomiting, threatened abortion.

拓展模块

砂仁作为一种较为温和的草药，在中国的应用已经有 1300 多年的历史。广东省阳春市是砂仁的道地产区，这里所产的砂仁叫作春砂仁，因此阳春市享有"中国春砂仁之乡"的美誉。砂仁气香浓郁，味辛辣，李时珍在《本草纲目》中就记载了"春砂仁"具有"健胃、化滞、消食、安胎"等功效。同时，砂仁也是一种芳香性辛香调味食品，是火锅、卤料中常用的一种香料，被收载于《既是食品又是药品的物品名单》。

需要注意的是，在煎药的时候，砂仁一定要后下。也就是说，在其他药物快要煎好时，再将砂仁投入，煎 5 到 10 分钟即可。因为砂仁中的主要成分是挥发油，在高温下容易挥发或被破坏，这样的话就会降低药效，甚至失去药效。

虽然砂仁属于温性的一种中药，副作用不是很明显，但也不能长期过量吃。尤其阴虚有热的人和妇女产后不宜食用，患有肺结核、支气管扩张等病症者也不宜服用。

Related information

As a mild herb, Sharen has been used in China for more than 1300 years. Yangchun City of Guangdong Province is the production region of the best Sharen. And Sharen produced here is called Chun Sharen. Therefore, Yangchun City enjoys the reputation of "the hometown of Chun Sharen in China". Sharen has strong aroma and spicy taste. Li Shizhen recorded in the *Compendium of Materia Medica* that it has the functions of "strengthening stomach, removing stagnation, promoting digestion and preventing miscarriage". At the same time, Sharen is also a kind of aromatic spicy seasoning food, which is a common spice in hot pot and thick gravy. It is included in List of Items That Are both Food and Medicine.

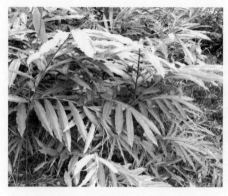
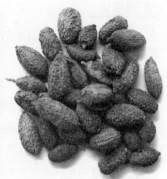

It should be noted that when decocting, Sharen must be "decocted later". That is to say, when other medicines are almost done, add Sharen into the pot and decoct all the medicines together for 5 to 10 minutes. Because the main component of Sharen is volatile oil which is likely to volatilize or be destroyed at high temperature, if so, its efficacy will be reduced or even lost.

Although Sharen is a kind of Chinese medicine with a warm nature and its side effects are not obvious, it cannot be overeaten for a long time. Besides, it is not suitable especially for people with yin deficiency and heat, or postpartum women, or patients with tuberculosis, bronchiectasis, etc.

故事模块

传说很久以前，广东的阳春县发生了一次范围较广的牛瘟，病死了许多耕牛，唯独蟠龙镇金花坑附近的耕牛不仅没有染病，反而身强力壮。这到底是怎么回事呢？当地几个老农便询问牧童们每天在哪里放牛，耕牛都吃些什么草。牧童们回答说他们在金花坑放牛，牛很喜欢吃这里生长的一种草。老农们听后，就和牧童们一起来到金花坑，看见那里漫山遍野生长着这种长得很像姜的植物，他们就采了一些回去熬药给牛治病，果然治好了。于是人们就想，既然这种草可治牛瘟，是否也能给人治病？通过实践后，人们发现这种草药对脾胃虚寒、泄泻呕吐等症也有很好的效果。这种草药就是阳春砂仁。

Story

Legend has it that a long time ago, a terrible cattle-plague struck Yangchun County in Guangdong Province and killed many farming cattle. Only the farming cattle near Jinhua Pit in Panlong Town were not infected; instead, they were still as strong as before. Several local farmers wondered why, and asked the shepherds where the cattle were grazing and what grass they were eating. The shepherds replied that they were herding cattle in the Jinhua Pit where the cattle liked eating a kind of grass growing here. After hearing this, the farmers went there together. They saw this kind of ginger-like plant growing in the wild all over the mountains. They picked some of this plant to treat their cattle and amazingly the cattle were cured. Therefore, people thought, "Since this grass can cure the cattle, will it cure people?" Through experiments, people found that this herbal medicine has a good effect on some syndromes such as deficiency-cold of spleen and stomach, diarrhea and vomiting. This herb is Yangchun Sharen.

（五）皮类 / Bark

杜仲
Duzhong / Eucommia Bark / Cortex Eucommiae

知识模块

来源：杜仲科（Eucommiaceae）植物杜仲 *Eucommia ulmoides* Oliv. 的干燥树皮。

产地：主产于湖北、四川、贵州、云南等地。

本草始载：始载于东汉《神农本草经》。

功效：补肝肾，强筋骨，安胎，降血压。

主治：治疗腰膝酸软、筋骨无力、妊娠胎动不安、高血压。

Basic knowledge

Origin: The dry bark of *Eucommia ulmoides* Oliv. belonging to the family Eucommiaceae.

Location: Duzhong is mainly produced in Hubei, Sichuan, Guizhou, and Yunnan provinces, etc.

First recorded in: *Shenong's Classic of Materia Medica* of the Eastern Han Dynasty

Efficacy: Nourishing liver and kidney, strengthening tendons and bones, preventing abortion, lowering blood pressure.

Indications: Soreness and pain in lumbar and knees, weak tendons and bones, threatened abortion, and hypertension.

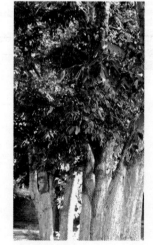

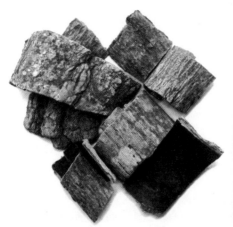
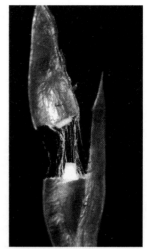

掰断果实后的白色拉丝

拓展模块

　　杜仲是我国特有的树种。如果把杜仲的叶、皮和果实折断，会看到有白丝相连，这白丝的主要成分就是橡胶，所以杜仲也是我国未来橡胶工业的潜在原料。除此之外，杜仲树形优美，在我国分布广泛，非常适合应用到城市绿化中作行道树。杜仲和杜仲叶都被收载于《可用于保健食品的物品名单》。杜仲叶可以加工成杜仲茶，用于降血压和血脂。

Related information

　　Duzhong tree / Eucommia tree is a unique species in China. If you break its leaf, bark or fruit, you will see the white stretchy substance, and the main ingredient in it is rubber. Therefore, it is a potential raw material for the future rubber industry in China. In addition, it has beautiful shapes and is an important tree in urban forestry. Both Duzhong bark and Duzhong leaf are included in List of Items That

Can Be Used as Health Food. For example, Duzhong leaves can be processed into Duzhong tea which can help lower blood pressure and blood lipids.

故事模块

杜仲这个名字看起来像不像一个人名？其实有几味中药的名字确实和人名有关系，比如刘寄奴这味药的名字相传来自南朝刘宋的开国皇帝刘裕（小名寄奴），徐长卿这味药的名字据说来自唐代的一位民间医生。那么杜仲呢？

相传古时有位叫杜仲的大夫，他有腰腿酸痛的老毛病。有一天他进山采药，偶然间看到一棵粗壮挺拔的参天大树，他发现树皮里有像"筋"一样的白丝。他觉得这棵大树真是不同寻常，就想人若吃了这树皮的"筋骨"，会不会也像这树一样筋骨强健？于是，他下决心亲自尝试。结果服用几天后，他的腰腿也不觉得酸痛了，坚持长期服用后，他不仅身轻体健，最后竟然得道成仙而去。因此后来人们就将这种树叫作"杜仲"。

这个故事并非凭空杜撰出来的，李时珍在《本草纲目》中记载："昔有杜仲服此得道，因以名之。"虽然这带有神话色彩，但也印证了李时珍所记载的杜仲的功效——"坚筋骨，治肾虚腰痛，久服，轻身耐老"。

Story

Do you think the name of Duzhong looks like a person's name? In fact, several Chinese herbal medicines do have the names of people. For example, the Chinese name of Liujinu (diverse wormwood herb) is said to come from Liu Yu (whose childhood name was Jinu), the founding emperor of Song State (420-479) of the Southern Dynasty (420-589). The Chinese name of Xuchangqing (paniculate swallowwort root) is said to come from a doctor in the Tang Dynasty. What about Duzhong?

According to legend, there was a doctor named Du Zhong in ancient times. He had been suffering from soreness and pain in his lumbar and knees. One day, while he was collecting medicinal herbs in the mountains, he happened to see a tall and strong tree, and found some white silk like "tendons" in the bark of the tree. He said to himself, "How unusual it is! If people took its bark, would they become as strong as the tree?" So he made up his mind to try it himself. As a result, after a few days, his lumbar and legs did feel much better. After taking it for a long time, he was not only healthy, but eventually he was able to become immortal. Therefore, people called this tree "Duzhong".

This story is not fabricated out of thin air. Li Shizhen recorded in his *Compendium of Materia Medica*: "In the past, a man named Du Zhong took it and became immortal. That's why the tree got its name." Although this description is mythical, it reflects the efficacy of Duzhong recorded by Li Shizhen—"(It can) strengthen the tendons and bones, and cure backache caused by kidney deficiency. People will have a flexible body and delay their senility if taking it for a long time."

（六）茎木类 / Stem and Wood

沉香
Chenxiang / Chinese Eaglewood/
Lignum Aquilariae Resinatum

知识模块

来源： 瑞香科（Thymelaeceae）植物白木香 *Aquilaria sinensis* (Lour.) Gilg 及沉香 *A. agallocha* Roxb. 含树脂的心材。

产地： 白木香主产于广东、广西、海南等地。沉香主产于印度尼西亚、马来西亚、越南、柬埔寨等东南亚国家。

本草始载： 始载于魏晋时期《名医别录》。

功效： 行气止痛，温中降逆，纳气平喘。

主治： 治疗寒凝气滞疼痛，胃寒呕逆以及虚喘证等。

Basic knowledge

Origin: The resinous heartwood of *Aquilaria sinensis* (Lour.) Gilg and *A. agallocha* Roxb. belonging to the family Thymelaeceae.

Location: *Aquilaria sinensis* (Lour.) Gilg is mainly produced in Guangdong Province, Guangxi Zhuang Autonomous Region and Hainan Province of China. *A. agallocha* Roxb. is mainly produced in Southeast Asian countries such as Indonesia, Malaysia, Viet Nam, Cambodia, etc.

First recorded in: *Ming Yi Bie Lu* (*Miscellaneous Records of Famous Physicians*) of Wei-Jin Period.

Efficacy: Regulating qi and alleviating pain, warming middle energizer and descending adverse qi, improving qi reception and relieving dyspnea.

Indications: Pain caused by cold congelation and qi stagnation, vomiting and hiccup due to stomach cold, and dyspnea of deficiency type, etc.

拓展模块

沉香非常名贵，好的沉香可以说是价值连城。除药用外，它广泛用于香料、香水、熏香中。沉香主要产自中国的两广、海南以及东南亚的一些国家，如越南、老挝、缅甸、柬埔寨、泰国，以及印尼、马来西亚、菲律宾等。

你知道沉香是怎么产生的吗？正常情况下沉香树的心材是没有香味的，当沉香树受伤后，真菌侵入伤口，使其薄壁组织细胞内的淀粉产生一系列的化学变化，最后形成香脂，凝结于木材内。这也是沉香树在漫长的自然进化过程中形成的一种自我保护措施。

为了加速结香，人工干预是必不可少的。常见的方法就是刀劈斧砍，以及钻洞等方式人为对沉香树（或白木香）制造创伤，以促进其结香。

Related information

Chenxiang is very valuable, and the top-grade Chenxiang is even invaluable. It is also widely used in perfumes, fragrance and incense besides medicinal uses. It is mainly produced in Guangdong, Guangxi and Hainan of China, and some Southeast Asian countries such as Vietnam, Laos, Myanmar, Cambodia, Thailand, and Indonesia, Malaysia, the Philippines and so on.

Do you know how it is produced? Under normal circumstances, the heartwood of aquilaria trees is odorless. When the tree is injured, the fungus invades the wound and thus the starch in its parenchyma cells

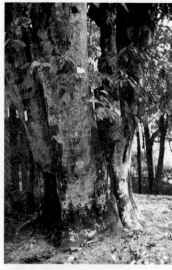

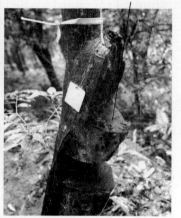

浸有黑色树脂的木材

一棵上千年的白木香树　　　　　斧砍"开香门"

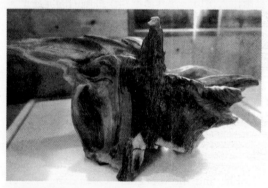

这块沉香价值百万

will have a series of chemical changes. Therefore, aromatic resin is finally produced and it condenses in the wood. This is the self-protection of aquilaria trees developed during the natural evolution.

In order to speed up the formation of resin, manual intervention is essential. The common method is to chop the tree with knives or axes, or drill holes in the tree to create wounds to promote the formation of Chenxiang.

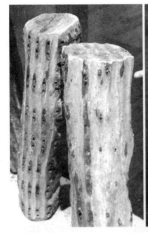
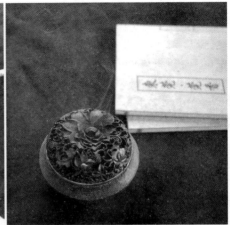

钻洞结香　　　　　　做成高档熏香

故事模块

　　我国古代人们很早就将沉香视为珍贵之物。《三国演义》中有记载，关羽败走麦城被孙权杀死，孙权命人把关公首级献给曹操，曹操命人用沉香雕成他的身躯，并以王侯之礼安葬他。梁代陶弘景《名医别录》中把沉香列为中药里的"上品"。隋代时，沉香又被皇室和皇族大量使用在饰品及建筑装潢上，比如隋炀帝每到除夕就会焚烧沉香数十车，方圆数十里都能闻到香味。唐宋明清等后世各朝中，沉香都受到极大推崇，有钱人家用它制作家具和亭台楼阁，或者用来制茶、焚香。

　　当然，沉香的医用价值不可忽略，有记载古时有个酒店老板叫刘三，一天早上起来，他面色发黑，就像用煤灰抹了脸一样。镇上郎中诊断说这可是不治之症，一月内必死无疑。从此刘三精神消沉，家人恐慌。一天，一位江湖郎中路过，询问过详情后，郎中判断他是上茅厕时受到了浊气的影响，于是让他买来沉香，并在蚊帐内焚香蒸熏祛除体内秽气。果然刘三的症状渐渐消失，第二天就恢复如初。可见良医能够辨证论治、对症下药从而治病救人。

Story

People in ancient China regarded Chenxiang as a highly valuable thing. In *Romance of the Three Kingdoms*, Guan Yu was defeated in Maicheng, and then he was killed by Sun Quan who then dedicated the chopped-off head of Guan Yu to Cao Cao. Cao Cao, who appreciated Guan Yu very much, ordered people to carve the body with Chenxiang wood for Guan Yu and then held a grand funeral for him. Tao Hongjing, a famous doctor in Liang Dynasty (502-557), listed Chenxiang as a top grade Chinese herbal medicine in *Miscellaneous Records of Famous Physicians*. In the Sui Dynasty (581-618 or 619), Chenxiang was used extensively by the imperial family and the royal family in ornaments and architectural decoration. For example, Emperor Yang of the Sui Dynasty burned dozens of carriages of Chenxiang on New Year's Eve and the fragrance spread as far as over tens of miles. In later dynasties like Tang, Song, Ming and Qing Dynasties, Chenxiang was highly popular among the wealthy people who used it to make furniture and pavilions, or to make tea and incense.

Of course, the medical value of Chenxiang cannot be ignored. There is a story of an ancient hotel owner called Liu San. One morning, his found his face had turned black, as if his face was covered with coal ashes. The doctor in the town diagnosed that this was an incurable disease and he would die within a month. Therefore, Liu San and his family were scared and depressed. However, one day a quack doctor was passing by. After asking for details, this doctor judged that Liu San was affected by the filthy air when he went to the toilet. So he asked Liu San to buy some Chenxiang, and then burn the Chenxiang in the bed-curtain so that the incense could remove the bad odor in his body. Sure enough, Liu San's symptoms gradually disappeared and he recovered the second day. It can be seen that good doctors can prescribe the right medicine based on syndrome differentiation to treat the patients.

鸡血藤

Jixueteng / Suberect Spatholobus Stem / Caulis Spatholobi

知识模块

来源：豆科（Leguminosae）植物密花豆 *Spatholobus suberectus* Dunn 干燥藤茎。

产地：主产于广东、广西、海南及云南等地。

本草始载：始载于清代《本草备要》。

功效：补血，活血，通络。

主治：治疗血虚月经不调，风湿痹痛，麻木瘫痪等。

Basic knowledge

Origin: The dry stem of *Spatholobus suberectus* Dunn belonging to the family Leguminosae.

Location: Jixueteng is mainly produced in Guangdong Province, Guangxi Zhuang Autonomous Region, Hainan Province, and Yunnan Province, etc.

First recorded in: *Ben Cao Bei Yao* (*Essentials of Matea Medica*) of the Qing Dynasty.

Efficacy: Replenishing blood, activating blood circulation, dredging collaterals.

Indications: Irregular menstruation due to blood deficiency, rheumatic arthralgia, numbness and paralysis, etc.

拓展模块

鸡血藤的茎被切断以后，会慢慢渗出鲜红色的汁液，看起来很像鸡

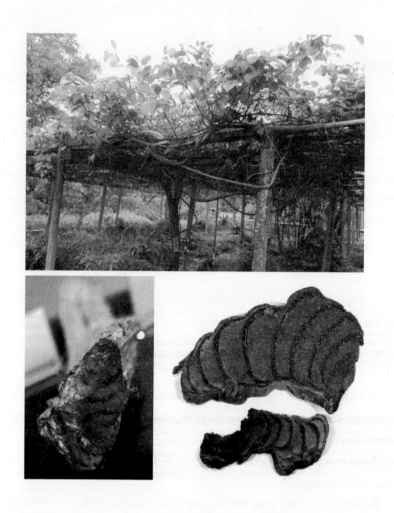

血，因此，人们称它为鸡血藤。由于其漂亮的棕红色，鸡血藤也可被制作成手镯供人佩戴。鸡血藤植物用途广泛，可搭花架或者是做盆景，都有很好的观赏效果。它的藤和根可供药用，有行气、活血、舒筋、活络等功效。鸡血藤也是治疗癌症的常用中草药，尤其是治疗癌症引起的贫血的要药。

Related information

When you cut open the stems of Jixueteng, you will see bright red juice gradually oozing from the wound. This juice looks like chicken blood, and that's why it is called Jixueteng (which literally means chicken blood vine). Because of its beautiful brown-red color, it can also be made into bracelets. Jixueteng is widely used in daily life. For example, it can be made into flower rack or bonsai, which has a good viewing effect. Its vine and root can be used for medicinal purposes, such as promoting qi, activating blood circulation, relaxing tendons, and so on. It is also a Chinese herbal medicine commonly used for cancer treatment, especially for anemia caused by cancer.

故事模块

古时有一后生叫李富，给财主放牛，由于日久劳作，患上了手足麻木的毛病。狠心的财主不愿给他花钱治病，便把他赶出家门。他只得上山采药，以卖药为生。李富非常善良乐于助人，遇到穷人生病没钱看病，他还会无私地赠药。

一天，李富采药很晚，在朦胧的月光下，他枕在一根藤上不知不觉地睡着了，还做了一个奇怪的梦，梦见自己喝了一只公鸡的血。醒来时已经黎明，他抬头望去，只见这根藤被他压断的地方流出像血液一样的红色液体，原来梦中喝的公鸡血就是这根藤的汁液。他感到喝了藤的汁液后身体舒畅，于是就每天砍一段藤条回家煮水喝。时间长了，他全身麻木、酸疼的症状全部消退。慢慢地，很多类似的病人也被这种药治愈。由于这种藤的汁液如同鸡血一般，人们便把这味药叫鸡血藤。

Long ago, there was a young cowherd named Li Fu. He worked for a landlord. His limbs became numb because of years of hard work. The landlord didn't want to spend any money on him, and then drove him out. He had no choice but to collect and sell medicinal herbs in the mountains for a living. Li Fu was kind-hearted and willing to help other people. When he met the poor who had no money to see a doctor, he just gave them his medicine for free.

One day, he was collecting herbs late into the night. In the dim moonlight, he leaned his head on the vine and fell asleep unconsciously. He had a strange dream that he drank the blood of a rooster. When he woke up, it was already dawn. Looking up, he saw that some blood-like liquid was dripping from the broken vine. It turned out that the rooster's blood that he drank in his dream was actually this red liquid from the vine. He felt rather comfortable after drinking the liquid, so from then on, he cut a piece of vine and boiled water to drink every day. Gradually his symptoms of numbness and soreness all disappeared. Later, many patients with similar symptoms were cured. Because the color of this vine is like rooster blood, people call this herb "Jixueteng" (which means the vine of rooster blood).

（七）其他类 / Other

芦荟
Luhui / Aloe

知识模块

来源： 百合科（Liliaceae）植物库拉索芦荟 *Aloe barbadensis* Miller、好望角芦荟 *Aloe ferox* Miller 或其他同属植物叶的汁液浓缩干燥物。

产地： 原产于非洲、美洲等地，现我国南方地区有引种。

本草始载： 始载于唐代《药性论》。

功效： 泻热通便，清肝热，驱蛔虫。

主治： 治疗热结便秘、小儿疳积，外治湿癣。

Basic knowledge

Origin: The dried concentrated leaf juice of *Aloe barbadensis* Miller, *Aloe ferox* Miller and other species belonging to the same genus of the family Liliaceae.

Location: Luhui is native to Africa and America. It has been introduced and planted in South China.

First recorded in: *Yao Xing Lun* (*Treatise on Herb Property*) of Tang Dynasty.

Efficacy: Purging heat and relaxing bowels, clearing liver-heat, expelling ascarid.

Indications: Heat-type constipation, children's malnutrition, acute eczema or dermatitis.

拓展模块

芦荟被载于《可用于保健食品的物品名单》。芦荟制品被广泛应用于食品、美容、保健、医药等领域。但芦荟也具有一定毒性，孕妇、婴幼儿不宜食用。普通人每日食用芦荟制品也不宜过多，否则轻者出现恶心、呕吐、腹泻等症状，重者可引起急性肾炎。

芦荟在我们生活中也有许多其他作用。比如，用芦荟叶中的胶质涂在脸上，会有保湿的作用。牙疼时可以把芦荟肉放在痛牙上轻轻咬住，大约 1～2 小时疼痛就会减轻。此外，烫伤时如果烫伤不严重，可以先凉水冲烫伤处，再覆上芦荟肉，用纱布固定，每天更换 2 次，会缓解疼痛，而且伤口恢复好后也不容易留疤。

Related information

Luhui is included in List of Items That Can Be Used as Health Food. Luhui products are widely used in food, beauty culture, health care, medicine and other fields. But Luhui also has certain toxicity. Pregnant

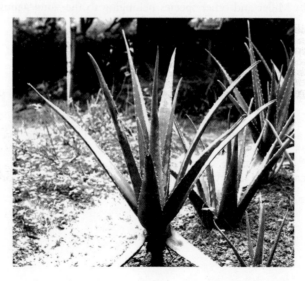

women and infants had better not take aloe. Even the ordinary people should not take too much of it. Otherwise, people might get poisoned. Those who are mildly poisoned might have symptoms such as nausea, vomiting, diarrhea and so on, and those who are severely poisoned can have acute nephritis.

Luhui has many magical effects in our life. For example, if you apply the gelatin of its leaves on your face, it will help keep skin moist. When you have toothache, you can put some meat of Luhui on your bad tooth and bite it lightly. The pain will be reduced in about 1~2 hours. In addition, if you get scalded not too seriously, you can first wash the scald with cold water, then covered it with Luhui meat, fix it with gauze, and change it twice a day, this will ease the pain, and the wound is unlikely to leave a scar after recovery.

故事模块

芦荟的药用价值很早就为人熟知。唐代著名诗人刘禹锡不仅在文学方面有着非凡的造诣，而且对医学也颇有研究，还曾经编撰过一本名为《传信方》的医书，书中记载了他少时生病的一次经历。刘禹锡少年时曾患癣疾，从脖子开始，慢慢地蔓延到耳朵，奇痒难忍，试过很多药都没什么效果，反而更厉害了。偶然间他来到楚州，遇到一位药商教他用芦荟和炙甘草混合在一起敷在患处，结果他用药之后很快就痊愈了。

除了医用价值，芦荟在美容方面也是众所周知的佳品，早在 2000多年前的亚历山大帝国，芦荟既是治疗日晒斑、溃疡、蚊虫叮咬、皮炎的良药，也是女性美容的圣品。传说并称"东方三大美女的"埃及艳后克利奥帕特拉、日本的小野小町及中国的杨贵妃都用芦荟保养皮肤。

1945 年美国在日本投下两颗原子弹，大批幸存者皮肤被核辐射灼伤，据说有人用芦荟涂抹伤口，愈合又快又好，不留瘢痕。

The medicinal value of Luhui has been known since ancient time. Liu Yuxi, a famous poet of the Tang Dynasty, has not only made great achievements in literature, but also done a lot of research about medicine. He has compiled a medical book titled *Chuan Xin Fang* in which he recorded one of his personal experiences. When he was a teenager, he suffered from eczema which started on his neck and later spread to his ears. The itching was really unbearable. He tried many medicines but all these medicines were useless and made him more painful instead. When he came to a place called Chuzhou, a pharmacist taught him to mix Luhui with roasted Gancao and apply the ointment to the affected area. Amazingly, he recovered soon.

Luhui is also a well-known beauty product. As early as 2000 years ago, in the Empire of Alexander the Great, it was not only used to treat sunburn, ulcers, insects and mosquitoes stings, dermatitis, but also used by women to keep their beauty. Legend has it that the so-called "three most beautiful women in the Orient"-Cleopatra of Egypt, Ono no Komachi of Japan, and Yang Yuhuan of China-all used Luhui for skin care.

In 1945, the United States dropped two atomic bombs in Japan, and a large number of survivors had their skin burned by nuclear radiation. It is said that some people applied Luhui on the wounds, and their wounds were healed quickly without leaving scars.

二、真菌类 / Fungus medicine

　　真菌是一种原始的真核生物。真菌的营养生长阶段主要以菌丝形式存在，不含叶绿素和其他光合色素，以异养方式（比如腐生和寄生）吸收寄主的营养。繁殖阶段会形成各种形态的菌丝体。生活中常见的蘑菇和酵母菌等就属于这一家族。常用的真菌类中药有冬虫夏草、灵芝、茯苓等等。

Fungi are primitive eukaryotes. The vegetative growth stage of fungi mainly exists in the form of hyphae, which does not contain chlorophyll and other photosynthetic pigments. Therefore, the fungi absorb the nutrition of the host in heterotrophic ways (such as saprophytic and parasitic). During the reproductive stage, various forms of mycelia are formed. Mushrooms and yeasts commonly seen in daily life belong to this family. The commonly used fungus medicines include Dongchongxiacao, Lingzhi, and Fuling and so on.

冬虫夏草

Dongchongxiacao / Chinese Caterpillar Fungus / Cordyceps Sinensis

＼ 知识模块

来源： 麦角菌科（Clavicipitaceae）真菌冬虫夏草菌 *Cordyceps sinensis* (Berk.) Sacc. 的子座及其寄主蝙蝠蛾科昆虫蝙蝠蛾 *Hepialus armoricanus* Oberthur. 幼虫尸体的复合体。

产地： 主产于四川、青海、西藏、甘南等地区。

本草始载： 始载于清代《本草从新》。

功效： 补肺益肾，止血，化痰。

主治： 治疗久咳虚喘，痨嗽咳血，阳痿遗精，腰膝酸痛。

＼ Basic knowledge

Origin: The complex of stroma of *Cordyceps sinensis* (Berk.) Sacc. belonging to the family Clavicipitaceae and the corpse of its host-*Hepialus armoricanus* Oberthur belonging to the family Hepialoidea.

Location: Dongchongxiacao is mainly produced in Sichuan Province, Qinghai Province, Tibet Autonomous Region, and south of Gansu Province, etc.

First recorded in: *Ben Cao Cong Xin* (*New Compilation of Materia Medica*) of the Qing Dynasty.

Efficacy: Tonifying lung and kidney, stopping bleeding, resolving phlegm.

Indications: Chronic cough, dyspnea of deficiency type, tuberculosis cough and hemoptysis, impotence, spermatorrhea, soreness and pain in lumbar and knees.

拓展模块

冬虫夏草属于藏药。它既名贵又奇异罕见，从地面上看它像一棵草，但挖出来后它的根却是一条虫。实际上它既不是草也不是虫，而是一种昆虫与寄生真菌的结合体。"虫"是受寄生真菌感染而死亡的虫草蝙蝠蛾幼虫的尸体，因为这种幼虫冬天生活在冻土中，所以叫"冬虫"；"草"是寄生在虫子身上的虫草真菌子座，形似草，因为它在夏天钻出地面，因此称为"夏草"。由于冬虫夏草生于高海拔恶劣环境中，且采收时间有限，所以野生产量很低，加之目前尚不能人工种植冬虫夏草，这就导致了它的价格非常昂贵。

冬虫夏草是我国民间传统的名贵滋补药材，与人参和鹿茸一起并称"中国三大补药"，有较高的营养价值，可以增强人的体质和免疫力，还能滋补肺肾，通常取 3 克至 10 克煎煮或泡水服用，也可泡酒、煲汤、煮粥服用，比如虫草老鸭汤。

Related information

Dongchongxiacao is a kind of Tibetan medicine. It is rare and precious. It looks like a grass above the ground, but when it is dug out, its root is actually a worm. In fact, it is neither a grass nor a worm, but a combination of worm and parasitic fungi. The "worm" is the corpse of Hepialus armoricanus Oberthu which dies of infection caused by parasitic fungi. It is called "Dong Chong / winter worm" because it lives in frozen soil in winter. The "grass" is the stroma of Cordyceps Fungus parasitic in the worm. It looks like grass and emerges from the ground in summer, so it is called "Xia Cao / summer grass". Because Dongchongxiacao grows at high altitude and the harvesting time is quite limited, the yield of wild Dongchongxiacao is very low. In addition, this kind of medicine cannot be cultivated artificially at present. All these factors lead to its pretty high price.

Dongchongxiacao is a valuable traditional tonic medicine in China. It is also called "three tonics of China" together with Renshen (ginseng) and Lurong (velvet antler). With a high nutritional value, it can invigorate health and enhance immunity effectively, and nourish lung and kidney. People can use 3 to 10 grams of it to decoct or soak in water each time, and can also use it to make medicinal wine, soup or porridge, such as Dongchongxiacao stewed with duck.

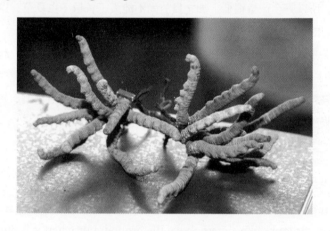

故事模块

　　关于冬虫夏草，藏族人民流传着不少美丽的传说。据说从前一个国王有两个儿子，小儿子聪明伶俐，很受老国王的喜欢。于是老大为了争夺王位就设下了毒计，想趁着弟弟到山上游玩的时候，将他杀死在山里。上仙得知了哥哥的阴谋，于是为了保护弟弟，便把他变成了一个虫子。老大一看弟弟不见了，只看到一只虫子，于是他施展魔法变成了一只山鹰，想去吃掉这个虫子，可是虫子很机灵地钻到了地里，并且长出一根草尾巴，把自己隐藏在草丛中。山鹰无可奈何，又气又急，结果掉下来摔死了。聪明的弟弟看破了红尘，不想再去继承王位当国王了，宁愿以自己的身躯为人们健康做出贡献。这件事感动了山神，山神就在他已变成虫子的身体里注入了长生不老的药，这种长着草的"虫子"就变成了能治病的冬虫夏草。从此，谁能勇敢而不避艰险地到冰峰雪岭去采挖虫草，那么它吃了以后也就可以延年益寿了。

Story

As for Dongchongxiacao, the Tibetan people have many beautiful legends. It is said that once a king had two sons. The king preferred his younger son because he was smart. In order to take the throne, the elder son planned to kill his younger brother when he was outing in the mountains. After knowing this conspiracy, a god in the heaven turned the younger brother into a worm in order to protect him. The elder brother didn't find his brother but saw a worm on the ground. So he used magic to turn himself into an eagle, trying to catch and eat the worm. But the worm shrewdly got into the ground, and then grew a grass tail, submerging itself in the sea of grasses. The eagle burned with a frenzy of rage. He dropped to the ground and died. The younger brother became disillusioned with the mortal world and he did not want to inherit the throne. He would rather sacrifice his own life to benefit all people's health. Touched by his choice, the mountain god put magic medicine into the body of the worm, and then it became Dongchongxiacao which could cure many diseases. From then on, those who are brave enough to climb to the icy and snowy peaks can prolong their life by eating Dongchongxiacao that they dig up there.

灵芝

Lingzhi / Glossy Ganoderma / Ganoderma

知识模块

来源： 多孔菌科（Polyporaceae）真菌灵芝（赤芝）*Ganoderma lucidum* (Leyss. ex Fr.) Karst. 或紫芝 *G. sinense* Zhao, Xu et Zhang 的干燥子实体。

产地： 赤芝主产于华东、西南及河北、山西、江西、广东、广西等地；紫芝主产于浙江、江西、湖南、广西、福建和广东等地。

本草始载： 始载于东汉《神农本草经》。

功效： 补气安神，止咳平喘。

主治： 治疗心悸气短，眩晕不眠，虚劳咳嗽。

Basic knowledge

Origin: The dry fruiting body of *Ganoderma lucidum* (Leyss. ex Fr.) Karst. (Chizhi) or *G. sinense* Zhao, Xu et Zhang (Zizhi) belonging to the family Polyporaceae.

Location: Chizhi (Red Lingzhi) is mainly produced in East and Southwest of China, as well as Hebei, Shanxi, Jiangxi, Guangdong provinces and Guangxi Zhuang Autonomous Region, etc.; Zizhi (Purple Lingzhi) is mainly produced in Zhejiang, Jiangxi, Hunan, Guangxi, Fujian and Guangdong provinces, etc.

First recorded in: *Shennong's Classic of Meteria Medica* of the Eastern Han Dynasty.

Efficacy: Benefiting qi for tranquillization, relieving cough and asthma.

Indications: Palpitation, shortness of breath, dizziness, insomnia, coughs due to deficiency.

拓展模块

灵芝含有灵芝多糖等物质，能够提高免疫力、抗癌防癌、护肝解毒、降血糖、抗衰老、改善神经衰弱，还能防治心血管病、防高血脂、中风等症。但天然灵芝较为稀少，远不能满足人们的需求，现在市场上的灵芝多以栽培为主，以赤芝栽培为多。由于目前灵芝栽培技术成熟，所以市场上的栽培灵芝价格很便宜，真正的物美价廉哦！

灵芝服用起来也很方便，可以先切成小块，然后泡水或煎水服用，也可以泡酒制成药酒。煮粥或炖汤时也可以加入适量的灵芝。此外，灵芝孢子常用于抗肿瘤，提高机体免疫力，也是一种不错的保健品。

Related information

Lingzhi contains ganoderma polysaccharides, and it can be very good for health if regularly used because it cannot only improve immunity, prevent cancer, protect liver, lower blood sugar, delay aging, improve neurasthenia, but also prevent cardiovascular disease, hyperlipidemia, stroke and other diseases. Wild Lingzhi is scarce and far from meeting people's needs. At present, most of Lingzhi in the market are artificially planted. The majority of them are Chizhi. With well-developed cultivation skills, the price of Lingzhi with good quality is not high. Cheap and fine, aren't they?

Lingzhi is also very convenient to take. You can cut Lingzhi into small pieces first, and then drink the water soaked or boiled with Lingzhi pieces. Lingzhi can also be made into medicinal wine. It can also be added to the porridge or soup. Besides, Lingzhi spore is commonly used to fight cancer and enhance immunity, and thus is also a good health care product.

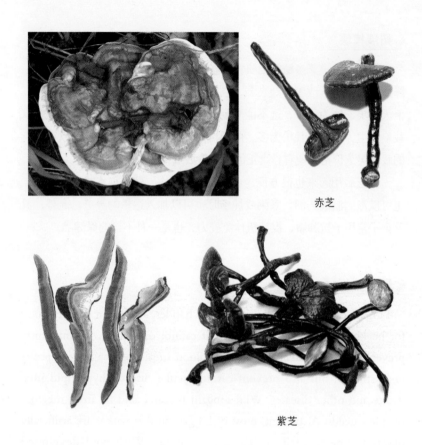

赤芝

紫芝

故事模块

　　在民间传说《白蛇传》中，白蛇白素贞修炼千年修得人形，与书生许仙互相爱慕结为夫妇。适逢中秋佳节，夫妇俩人喝了雄黄酒，白素贞就现出了白蛇的原型，竟然把许仙活活吓死了，白素贞就去昆仑山盗取仙草救活了丈夫。故事里面的"仙草"，据说就是灵芝。

　　灵芝自古以来被称为仙草，被认为是美好、吉祥、富贵和长寿的象征。关于它，有很多传说。月宫里的嫦娥因为灵芝而长生不老。武夷山彭祖活了760年，就是因为他服食了灵芝仙草。我国古代《山海经》中记载有这样一个传说：炎帝有一个最宠爱的女儿叫"瑶姬"，但不幸幼年夭折。炎帝怜惜爱女，封她为"姑瑶山神"，死后她的灵魂漂到姑瑶山上，变成了姑瑶山上的"瑶草"，即我们现今所称的灵芝。

　　当然，神话归神话，李时珍著的《本草纲目》和东汉时期《神农本草经》都有记载，这说明古代医药学家早已认识了灵芝的药用价值。灵芝的神奇疗效是毋庸置疑的，对心神不宁，失眠心悸，肺虚咳喘，虚劳短气，不思饮食都有非常好的疗效。

Story

In the folklore *Legend of the White Snake*, Bai Suzhen, a white snake, transformed into a beautiful woman after practicing Taoist magical arts for over one thousand years. She fell in love with Xu Xian, a scholar, and married him. On the Mid-Autumn Festival, the couple drank realgar wine, so Bai Suzhen revealed her true form, a large white snake. Xu Xian died of shock when he saw his wife was not human. Therefore, Bai Suzhen went to Kunlun Mountain and stole a magical herb to save her husband. The "magical herb" in the story is said to be Lingzhi.

Lingzhi is known as "magical herb" since ancient times. It is considered to be a symbol of goodness, auspiciousness, wealth and longevity. There are many legends about it. Chang'e, the goddess on the moon, was immortal because of Lingzhi. Peng Zu lived in Wuyi Mountain for 760 years, just because he took Lingzhi. There is a legend in *Classic of Mountains and Rivers* in ancient China that Emperor Yan had a favorite daughter named Yaoji, but unfortunately she died at her young age. Emperor Yan pitied his daughter and named her "Goddess of Guyao Mountain". After her death, her soul drifted to Guyao Mountain and turned into "Yao grass" on Guyao Mountain, which we now call Lingzhi.

Of course, this is just a myth. In *Compendium of Materia Medica* of Li Shizhen and *Shennong's Classic of Materia Medica* of the Eastern Han Dynasty, Lingzhi has already been recorded, which shows that ancient pharmacists have already known the medicinal value of Lingzhi. Its magical effect is indisputable. It has a very good effect on restlessness, insomnia, palpitation, asthma, exhaustion, shortness of breath, and poor appetite.

茯苓
Fuling / Indian Buead / Poria

来源: 多孔菌科（Polyporaceae）真菌茯苓 *Poria cocos* (Schw.) Wolf 的干燥菌核。

产地: 主产于安徽、云南、湖南、湖北、河南、贵州和四川等地。栽培茯苓主产于安徽大别山；野生茯苓主产于云南。

本草始载: 始载于东汉《神农本草经》。

功效: 利水渗湿，健脾，宁心安神。

主治: 治疗脾胃虚弱、水肿、小便不利和心神不宁。

Basic knowledge

Origin: The dried sclerotia of *Poria Cocos* (Schw.) Wolf belonging to the family Polyporaceae.

Location: Fuling is mainly produced in Anhui, Yunnan, Hunan, Hubei, Henan, Guizhou, and Sichuan provinces, etc. The cultivated Fuling is mainly produced in the Dabie Mountains in Anhui Province. The wild Fuling is mainly produced in Yunnan Province.

First recorded in: *Shenong's Classic of Materia Medica* of the Eastern Han Dynasty.

Efficacy: Inducing diuresis for clearing dampness, strengthening spleen, and tranquilizing mind.

Indications: Deficiency of spleen and stomach, edema, dysuria, restlessness.

拓展模块

　　茯苓具有健脾和胃、利水渗湿和宁心安神等作用，也有助于提高免疫力、控制血糖。它也是一种药食两用品种，被载入《既是食品又是药品的物品名单》中，既是传统中药，也是一种常用食品原料。相传慈禧太后为了养生，就命御膳房用白面和茯苓粉制成"茯苓饼"。除了茯苓饼，她的日常保健药方中也多用到茯苓这味药材。现在，茯苓饼已不再是皇家的专用美食，而是老百姓常见的一种滋补性传统名点。除了做茯苓饼，茯苓也可以用来做糕点、煮粥和炖汤等，能起到很好的保健作用。

Related information

Fuling has the functions of invigorating the spleen and stomach, inducing diuresis for clearing dampness, and tranquilizing the mind. It is also helpful to improve immunity and control blood sugar. It can be used as both medicine and food, and has been included in List of Items That Are both Food and Medicine. It is not only a Chinese herbal medicine, but also a commonly used ingredient. According to legend, Empress Dowager Cixi ordered the imperial cooks to make

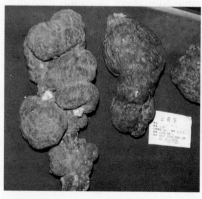 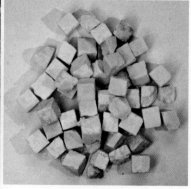

"Fuling Pie" with flour and Fuling powder in order to maintain health. Besides Fuling Pie, Fuling is also widely used in her daily health care prescriptions. Nowadays, Fuling Pie is no longer a royal delicacy, but a traditional nourishing snack for common people. Besides Fuling Pie, Fuling can also be used to make cakes, porridge, soup and so on, which can be very beneficial for people's health.

故事模块

相传成吉思汗在率军作战时，小雨连绵不断地下了好几个月，大部分将士染上了风湿病，眼看着就要兵败，成吉思汗十分着急。后来，有几个士兵因偶尔服食了茯苓，风湿病得以痊愈，成吉思汗听闻此事大喜，他急忙派人到盛产茯苓的湖北省罗田县运来大批茯苓给将士们吃，兵将们吃后风

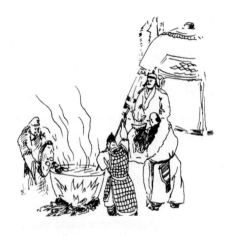

湿病好了起来，茯苓治疗风湿病的神奇功效也被广为传诵。

虽然上述故事的真实性无从考证，但足见茯苓的祛湿的功效早已被认可。北宋著名的文学家苏辙年少时体弱多病，夏则脾不胜食，秋则肺不胜寒。在其 32 岁那年，在调养治病的过程中，食用茯苓一年，竟然旧疾痊愈，从此便专心研究药物养生。他认为，茯苓是补肾脾的养生珍品，久服能"安魂魄而定心志"。后来，他还把这段经历写进自己的文章《服茯苓赋》里，并推荐人们用茯苓祛病延年。

Story

Legend has it that when Genghis Khan was leading his army in the battle, the light rain continued for several months. Most of the soldiers got rheumatism. Seeing the upcoming defeat, Genghis Khan was very anxious. Later, a few soldiers recovered from rheumatism by accidentally taking Fuling. After hearing about this, Genghis Khan was overjoyed. He hurriedly sent people to Luotian County of Hubei Province, a place rich in Fuling, to transport a large amount of Fuling for the soldiers. After taking Fuling, the soldiers got better, and the miraculous effect of Fuling in treating rheumatism was widely spread.

Although the authenticity of the above story cannot be verified, it can be seen that the effect of Fuling has been recognized long before. Su Zhe, a famous writer in the Northern Song Dynasty (960−1127), was weak and sick when he was young. In summer, he had no appetite due to spleen deficiency; in autumn, he couldn't bear the cool weather due to the weak lungs. However, at the age of 32, he was miraculously cured after taking Fuling for one year. From then on, he devoted himself to the study of health care with medicines. He believed that Fuling is a treasure that could nourish the kidney and spleen. It could "calm the soul and tranquilize the mind" if it was taken for a long time. Later, he wrote this personal experience into his essay "On Fuling", and recommended that people use Fuling for health care.

三、动物类 / Animal medicine

动物类中药占了整个中药的 10% 左右。根据入药部位不同，动物类中药包括：动物的全体入药，如一些小型节肢动物、环节动物等，如土鳖虫、全蝎、蜈蚣和地龙等；动物的皮肤分泌物或衍生物入药，如蟾酥、麝香和鹿茸等；动物组织及器官入药，如海螵蛸、阿胶和鸡内金等；动物的生理或病理产物入药，如牛黄、珍珠、蛇蜕和紫河车等；动物的排泄物入药，如五灵脂、蚕沙等（此类现在使用种类很少）。

Animal medicines account for about 10% of the Chinese herbal medicine. According to medicinal parts, animal medicines include the following categories: whole animal body, such as small arthropods or annelids, including woodlouse, scorpion, centipede and earthworm; the skin secretions or derivatives of animals, such as Chansu (toad venom), Shexiang (musk) and Lurong (velvet antler); animal tissues and organs, such as Haipiaoxiao (cuttlebone), Ejiao (donkey-hide gelatin) and Ji'neijin (chicken's gizzard-membrane); animal's physiological or pathological products, such as Niuhuang (bezoar), Zhenzhu (pearl), Shetui (snake slough) and Ziheche (human placenta); animal excretions (which are quite few), such as Wulingzhi (trogopterus dung) and Cansha (silkworm excrement).

全蝎
Quanxie / Scorpion / Scorpio

知识模块

来源：钳蝎科（Buthidae）动物东亚钳蝎 *Buthus martensii* Karsch 的干燥体。

产地：主产于河南、山东、河北和辽宁等地。

本草始载：始载于宋代《开宝本草》。

功效：息风止痉，攻毒散结，通络止痛。

主治：治疗中风，抽搐痉挛，半身不遂，风湿顽痹等。

Basic knowledge

Origin: The dry body of *Buthus martensii* Karsch belonging to the family Buthidae.

Location: Quanxie is mainly produced in Henan, Shandong, Hebei and Liaoning provinces, etc.

First recorded in: *Kai Bao Ben Cao (Materia Medica in Kai-Bao Reign)* of the Song Dynasty.

Efficacy: Calming endogenous wind to stop spasm, counteracting toxic pathogen and dissipating nodulation, dredging collateral and alleviating pain.

Indications: Stroke, convulsions, hemiplegia, rheumatism and so on.

拓展模块

活蝎尾部有毒腺，因此蝎子是民间俗称的"五毒"之首，在中医上是一种贵重的动物性药材，能治疗风湿痹痛、半身不遂和中风等病。它也是一种很好的食材。油炸或泡酒是较为常用的两种食用方法。油炸蝎子是山东的一道美食。做法是先将活蝎子放盐水中浸泡10分钟，之后放入烧热的油（或香油）中炸熟。炸好的蝎子，香酥可口，味道鲜美。全蝎也可以制作药酒，能起到一定的保健作用。但蝎子不可多吃，孕妇及过敏者慎用。

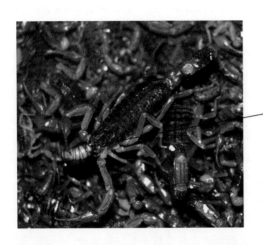
—— 一只正在吃食的蝎子

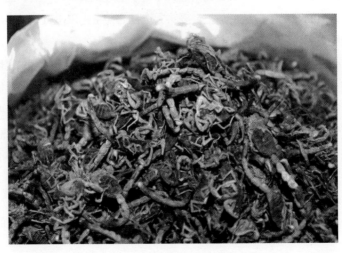

Related information

The tail of live scorpions contains toxic gland, so scorpion is commonly known as the first of the so-called "Wu Du" (the five toxic animals including scorpion, viper, gecko, centipede and toad); in Chinese herbal medicine, it is a valuable animal medicine that can treat rheumatism, arthralgia, hemiplegia, stroke and other diseases. It is also a good ingredient in daily diet. Fried scorpion and scorpion wine are two common methods. Fried Scorpion is a gourmet dish in Shandong. First drown live scorpions in salt water for 10 minutes, and then deep-fry them in hot oil or sesame oil. Fried Scorpion tastes crispy and very delicious. Scorpion can also be made into medicinal liquor which is beneficial for health care. However, scorpions should not be eaten too much at one time; besides, pregnant women and the people who are allergic to them should be cautious when taking scorpions.

故事模块

从前有个货郎，每天都到附近几个村子里赶集卖货。一天，他起得很早，就自己动手做饭，并把老婆头天洗好的菜拿进屋里做了一锅汤，吃饱喝足后他就挑起货担出门了。

他一口气走了十多里地，突然感到肚子里面像火烧一般，嘴里也像是有火一样渴得十分难受。可是，这一年天旱，到处都找不到水。货郎好不容易走到一座村庄，他推开第一家的院门，只有一个小孩在玩耍，这家也没有水。但货郎渴得口干舌燥，肚子里烧得难以忍受，他无意间在碗橱顶上发现一把茶壶，打开一看，壶里还有半壶陈茶。货郎不管三七二十一，对着壶嘴儿就喝。等到茶水灌进肚子，他觉得舒服多了，就谢过孩子，又挑上担子赶集去了。

再说货郎的老婆，天亮时爬起来吃饭，发现菜汤里竟有一条死的小毒蛇，心想货郎一定中毒了，说不定还没命了呢！她顾不上吃饭，一直跑到集市寻见丈夫。奇怪的是她丈夫竟像没事一样。她告诉了丈夫汤里有毒蛇，货郎看到自己没事非常纳闷，于是他们就来到那户人家，主人把茶壶捧出来，打开茶壶盖一看，里头有一只死蝎子和一条死蜈蚣。货郎心里一动，说："这就对啦！早晨喝了有蛇毒的汤，所以感到火烧心；后来又喝进有蝎毒、蜈蚣毒的茶，就没事了。这一定是毒能解毒呀！"

这是一段故事，不一定真有其事。不过，以毒攻毒还是有一定道理的。比如，后来，医生们从毒蛇的毒液中提取药素，可以治疗蛇伤和其他许多中毒的病症。蝎子也成了一味能治病救人的中药。

Story

Once upon a time, there was a street vendor who went to the countryside to sell goods every day. One day, he got up very early and cooked for himself. He made some soup with the vegetables his wife had washed the day before. After taking the soup, he carried the load of goods on his shoulder and went out.

He suddenly felt his stomach burning and he was very thirsty, but couldn't find any water due to the drought. Finally he managed to walk to a village. He pushed open the door of the first yard where only one child was playing. There was no water in the house either, but he was thirsty with a dry throat, and his stomach was burning heavily. Finally, he accidentally found a teapot on the top of the cupboard, with half pot of tea left in it. The vendor drank up the tea recklessly. He felt much better after drinking it. Then he thanked the child and picked up the load to go to the market.

The vendor's wife got up to have breakfast and found a small dead poisonous snake in the vegetable soup. She thought that her husband must have been poisoned. Maybe he was dead already! With no time to have breakfast, she immediately ran to the fair to look for her husband. Strangely enough, she found her husband was fine as usual. She told her husband about the poisonous snake in the soup. The vendor was very puzzled. So they went back to the house. The owner took the teapot out and removed the lid. There was a dead scorpion and a dead centipede in it. The vendor understood, and said, "That's right! In the morning, I drank the soup with snake venom, so my stomach burned so much. Later, I drank the tea with scorpion and centipede, but I am all right. The snake venom must have been detoxified by scorpion and centipede! "

This story is not necessarily true. However, it is reasonable to counteract one toxin with another. For example, doctors can extract useful medicine from the venom of vipers, which is used to treat snake wounds and many other poisoning symptoms. Scorpion is also a medicine that can cure many diseases.

海马
Haima / Seahorse / Hippocampus

知识模块

来源：海龙科（Syngnathidae）动物线纹海马 *Hippocampus kelloggi* Jordan et Snyder、刺海马 *H. histrix* Kaup、大海马 *H. kuda* Bleeker、三斑海马 *H. trimaculatus* Leach 或小海马（海蛆）*H. japonicus* Kaup 的干燥体。

产地：主产于广东、福建及台湾等地。我国其他沿海地区亦产。

本草始载：始载于唐代《本草拾遗》。

功效：补肾壮阳。

主治：治疗阳痿早泄、肾虚遗尿等症。

Basic knowledge

Origin: The dry body of *Hippocampus Kelloggi* Jordan et Snyder, *H. histrix* Kaup, *H. Kuda* Bleeker, *H. trimaculatus* Leach or *H. japonicus* Kaup belonging to the family Syngnathidae.

Location: Haima is mainly produced in Guangdong, Fujian, Taiwan provinces and other coastal areas of China.

First recorded in: *Ben Cao Shi Yi* (*A Supplement to Materia Medica*) of the Tang Dynasty.

Efficacy: Tonifying kidney and strengthening yang.

Indications: Impotence, premature ejaculation, enuresis due to kidney deficiency and other diseases.

海马是一种小型硬骨鱼，长相奇特，具有"马头、蛇尾、瓦楞身"的特征。海马最为奇特的是小海马是由海马爸爸"生"出来的。每年5至8月是海马的繁殖期，海马妈妈会把卵产在海马爸爸腹部的"育儿袋"里，然后接下来的孵化工作就交给海马爸爸负责了。等到海马宝宝孵化好后，才把宝宝们释放出来。所以，海马爸爸并不是真的把海马宝宝"生"出来，他只是起到了孵化海马宝宝的工作。当小海马遇到危险时，它们会钻到爸爸的育儿袋里。

海马能够强身健体、补肾壮阳、舒筋活络、消炎止痛、镇静安神和止咳平喘等，是一味不错的保健药。海马可以煲汤或泡酒。但是海马药性偏温，因此，孕妇及阴虚火旺者忌服。

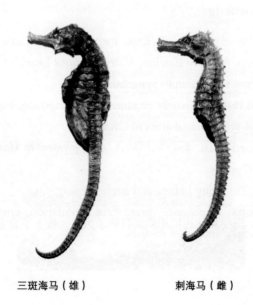

三斑海马（雄）　　　　　刺海马（雌）

Seahorse is a small bony fish with peculiar appearance characterized with "horse head, snake tail and corrugated body". The most peculiar feature of seahorses is that the seahorse babies are born by their father. During the breeding season every year from May to August, the female seahorse lays her eggs in the "brood pouch" on the ventral side of the tail of the male seahorse. Then incubation will be finished by the male seahorse. Then the male seahorse will release the babies into the water after they are fully developed. So the male seahorse doesn't really give birth to babies; actually, he is just responsible for incubation. When the babies meet dangers, they will hide in father's brood pouch.

Seahorse can make human body stronger, invigorate the kidney and strengthen yang, relax the tendons and collaterals, relieve inflammation and pain, calm the mind, and relieve cough and asthma, etc. It is a good health care medicine. It can be stewed with other ingredients or soaked in wine. However, the seahorse has a warm property, therefore, pregnant women and the patients with hyperactivity of fire due to yin deficiency should not take it.

故事模块

相传很久以前，在大海边住着一位勤劳的渔民名叫海生。他新婚不久后的一天，正在海上捕鱼，突然听到女子高呼救命的声音，海生连忙沿着声音寻去。原来是东海龙王的公主独自游玩时遇到了一条凶猛的大鱼要吃掉她。海生见状连忙用船桨打死了大鱼，救下了公主，公主十分感激海生的救命之恩，要送给海生珍贵的珠宝以作酬谢，但是善良的海生婉拒了公主。公主便允诺他以后有难时必会全力帮助他。

第二年春天，海生妻子分娩时遇上了难产，疼痛难忍，海生心急如焚，

225

正当他手足无措时，他突然想起来公主许下的承诺，便连忙来到海边寻到公主，恳请求公主帮忙。公主听闻，连忙命令巡海夜叉送药。

巡海夜叉牵过他那身材魁梧的坐骑海马，匆匆骑上就出发了。可是由于急于启程，他竟然忘记了喂马。海马跑了一阵，饥饿难忍，又不敢停蹄，忽然闻到夜叉的药袋里透出异香，便趁其不备，把药袋和药一口吞下。药入肚后，海马顿时精力充沛，于是就撒开四蹄，不一会儿就来到了海生家。这时候夜叉发现药袋不见了，又发现马嘴里有异香，断定药被马偷吃了，不禁大怒。

海马自知闯了大祸，转身就跑，逃进了礁石的缝隙中，不料却把身体给挤扁了。不过，海马知错就改，自己从岩缝中钻了出来，但四条腿和身子已经挤在了一起。因为海马吃了宝药，浑身都已成宝，当海马被带到海生家时，顿时满屋飘香，海生的妻子闻到药的香气，身子顿感轻松，"哇"的一声，孩子呱呱坠地。海生又请求公主让海马留在浅海近处，任其生长，以便能造福百姓。自此，海马就变成了现在看到的扁扁的模样，但也成了一味能治病救人的中药。

Story

According to the legend, once upon a time, there was a diligent fisherman named Haisheng. One day shortly after his marriage, he went fishing at sea. Suddenly he heard a woman's screaming "Help". It turned out to be the Princess of the Dragon King of the East China Sea. When she was hanging out alone, a fierce big fish tried to eat her. Haisheng killed the big fish with the oar and rescued the Princess. The Princess was grateful for him and tried to thank him with pearls in the Dragon Palace. However, Haishen refused her politely. The Princess promised that she would try her best to help him when he was in trouble in the future.

The next spring, Haisheng's wife suffered from difficult labor in childbirth and was in a great pain. While he was so anxious and didn't know what to do, he suddenly remembered the promise made by the Princess. So he went to the seaside and asked the Princess to help him. After knowing what happened to his wife, the Princess hastily ordered a yaksha to deliver medicine.

The yaksha mounted his seahorse which was tall and strong. But he was in such a hurry that he forgot to feed this seahorse. Therefore the seahorse ran for a while and became very hungry, but it dared not to stop. Suddenly, it smelled the odor in the medicine bag and swallowed the bag and medicine in one gulp. After taking the medicine, the seahorse instantly became energetic, and soon came to Haisheng's home. The yaksha found that the medicine bag had disappeared and a strange fragrance came from the horse's mouth. Obviously the medicine had been eaten by the horse, and he became very angry with the horse.

The seahorse knew he had made a huge mistake, so it turned around and ran away, escaping into the crevice of the reef and thus squashing its body. Then the seahorse got itself out of the crevice, but its four legs and body had been squeezed together. Because the seahorse took the treasure medicine, its whole body has become a treasure. When it was brought to Haisheng's home, the house immediately was filled with fragrance. After smelling it, Haisheng's wife felt a burst of relaxation and seconds later the baby was born. Haisheng asked the Princess to leave the flat seahorse in the shallow sea so as to help and benefit the common people. Since then, seahorses have become flat and also a precious medicine.

鹿茸

Lurong / Velvet Antler / Cornu Cervi Pantotrichum

知识模块

来源：鹿科（Cervidae）动物梅花鹿 *Cervus nippon* Temminck 或马鹿 *C. elaphus* Linnaeus 的雄鹿未骨化密生茸毛的幼角。前者称为"花鹿茸"，后者称为"马鹿茸"。

产地：花鹿茸主产于东北地区；马鹿茸主产于东北及西部地区。

本草始载：始载于东汉《神农本草经》。

功效：补肾壮阳、生精益血和补髓健骨。

主治：肾虚导致的头晕、耳聋、目暗、阳痿、滑精和宫冷不孕等症。

Basic knowledge

Origin: The hairy cartilaginous antlers of *Cervus nippon* Temminck, or *C. elaphus* Linnaeus belonging to the family cervidae. The former is called as "Hua Lurong / sika deer antler" and the latter is called as "Ma Lurong / red deer antler".

Location: Hua Lurong is mainly produced in Northeast of China; Ma Lurong is mainly produced in Northeast and West of China.

First recorded in: *Shenong's Classic of Materia Medica* of the Eastern Han Dynasty.

Efficacy: Tonifying kidney and strengthening yang, supplementing essence and blood, strengthening tendons and bones.

Indications: Lurong can treat many diseases caused by kidney deficiency such as dizziness, deafness, dim vision, impotence, spermatorrhea, infertility due to cold uterus, and so on.

拓展模块

　　鹿茸是我国东北的三宝之一（人参、貂皮和鹿茸）。梅花鹿和马鹿是我国产鹿茸的主要鹿种，尤其是梅花鹿的鹿茸最为名贵。鹿茸每年可以割两次。从 5 月份开始，公鹿生茸。生茸后经 56～58 天即可割茸。之后 10 天左右又开始重新生茸，等到鹿茸长至 50 天就要立即再次割茸。一定要注意鹿茸是没有骨化的嫩角，也就是要带茸毛，含血液，一旦鹿茸骨化就失去了其营养价值。

　　鹿茸可用于日常食疗保健，如可以用鹿茸片泡酒、煲汤和煮粥，或是磨成粉服用。鹿一身都是宝，除鹿茸外，鹿角（骨化的角）、鹿尾、鹿筋、鹿鞭、鹿胎、鹿血、鹿心和鹿油等均可入药或做滋补品服用。

Related information

Lurong is one of the three treasures (Renshen, mink fur and Lurong) in Northeast of China. Sika deer and red deer are the main deer species for Lurong in our country, and especially the antlers of sika deer are the most precious. Lurong can be cut twice each year. From May, the male deer start to grow velvet antlers. Antlers can be cut after 56−58 days. After 10 days or so, new antlers began to regenerate, and after 50 days, the velvet antlers should be cut again immediately. Lurong should be young antlers which are not ossified, in other words, they are hairy antlers with blood. Once they are ossified, their nutrition will be lost.

Lurong can be used in daily diet for health care. For example, Lurong slices can be made into medicinal wine, or cooked in soup and porridge, or ground into powder. The deer is a treasure all over its body. Besides velvet antlers, deer antlers (ossified antlers), deer tail, deer tendon, deep "whip" (dried penis and testicles of deer), deer fetus, deer blood, deer heart and deer oil can be used as medicine or tonic.

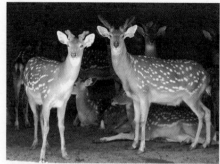
梅花鹿

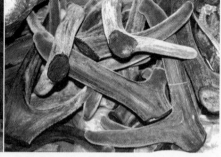
梅花鹿茸

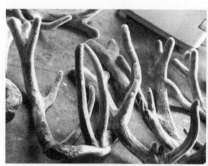
马鹿茸

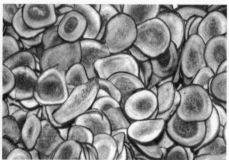
鹿茸片

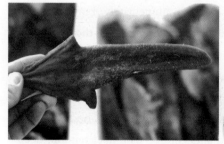
鹿尾

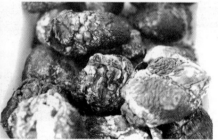
鹿心

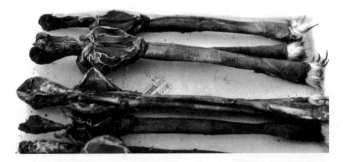

鹿鞭

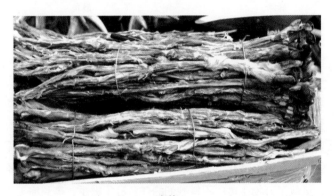

鹿筋

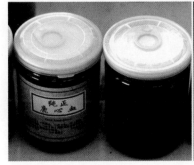

鹿心血

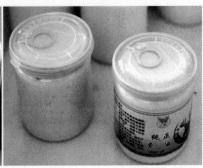

鹿油

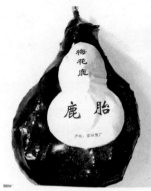
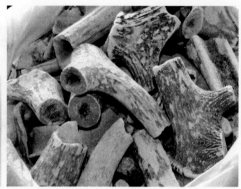

鹿胎　　　　　　　　　　　　鹿角

　　在长白山地区流传着一个美丽的传说：相传很久以前，关东的大地上没有一条大江大河，一到了旱季，生活在这里的动物们就没有水喝，饱受干旱的折磨。王母娘娘知道后十分同情这些动物，于是就派了七仙女降临凡间，她们凿开了长白山天池，流出的池水形成了奔流不息的松花江，拯救了万物生灵。不料她们的任务过于繁重，等到完工的时候，七仙女们都一个个地累倒了，已经没有力气飞起来了，如果她们不能按时返回天庭便会受到惩罚。正在这时，从森林中跑出来一只梅花鹿，来到仙女面前，只见它泪眼婆娑，猛地向石坨子撞去，撞断了头上的嫩角，然后口含鹿茸用鹿茸血去喂仙女饮用。得到了鹿茸的滋补，七仙女们转眼间就变得精神焕发，辞别这只梅花鹿后及时回到了天庭。

　　这个故事虽是虚构的，却也说明了鹿茸的神奇药效。鹿茸是自古以来人们用来强身健体的滋补佳品。清朝的乾隆皇帝就对鹿茸情有独钟。乾隆足足活了89岁，他经常服用的保健药品之一就是龟龄集，而龟龄集的一味重要药材就是鹿茸。

232

Story

There is a beautiful legend in the Changbai Mountains. It is said that a long time ago, there was no big river in the land of Northeast China. Animals living here had no water to drink in the dry season and suffered from drought. The Queen Mother in the Heavenly Palace was very sympathetic to these animals, so she sent seven fairies to the human world. They cut the Tianchi of Changbai Mountain, and the water flowing down from Tianchi formed into the Songhua River, which saved all living creatures. But unexpectedly, their task was so tiresome that the seven fairies were all exhausted and had no strength to fly by the time it was finished. If they could not fly back to the Heavenly Palace on time, they would be punished. Just then, a sika deer ran out of the forest and came to the fairies. It burst into a stone with tearful eyes, broke its tender antlers, and then fed the fairies with blood from the antler. Having been nourished by the antler blood, the seven fairies became energetic again quite soon, and then they returned to heaven in time after bidding farewell to the sika deer.

Although the story is fictional, it illustrates the magical efficacy of Lurong. Actually, it has always been a good tonic for people to strengthen their health since ancient times. Emperor Qianlong of the Qing Dynasty had a special preference for Lurong. He lived to the age of 89. One of the health medicines he often took was Guilingji, and one of its main ingredients is Lurong.

蜂蜜
Fengmi / Honey / Mel

来源：蜜蜂科（Apidae）昆虫中华蜜蜂 *Apis cerana* Fabricius 或意大利蜜蜂 *A. mellifera* Linnaeus 所酿的蜜。

产地：全国大部分地区均产，均为人工养殖生产。

本草始载：始载于东汉《神农本草经》。

功效：补脾益气，润燥，缓急止痛，解毒。

主治：治疗脾胃虚弱，肺燥咳嗽，肠燥便秘等。

Basic knowledge

Origin: The honey produced by *Apis cerana* Fabricius, or *A. mellifera* Linnaeus belonging to the family Apidae.

Location: It is produced in most parts of China, all by artificial culture.

First recorded in: *Shenong's Classic of Materia Medica* of the Eastern Han Dynasty.

Efficacy: Invigorating spleen and replenishing qi, moistening dryness, alleviating pain and detoxicating.

Indications: Spleen and stomach deficiency, cough due to dryness in lung, constipation due to dryness in intestines, etc.

蜂蜜自古以来被视作滋补强身的佳品，如今随着生活水平的提高更是备受人们的追捧。它被收载于《既是食品又是药品的物品名单》中。

蜂蜜是一种天然食品，具有润肺止咳、润肠通便、帮助睡眠、补充体力和快速醒酒等功效，长期食用可以为身体提供营养，还能调理身体各器官的功效，减少一些常见疾病的发生。此外，蜂蜜还常用作美容产品中，自己在家也可以用蜂蜜搭配蛋清、牛奶和橄榄油等材料自制面膜，效果很不错。除了蜂蜜，蜂胶、蜂蜡、蜂子、蜂蛹和蜂王浆等均可入药或作为保健品食用。

要注意冲泡蜂蜜水不能直接用沸水，否则会破坏蜂蜜里丰富的维生素和矿物质。而且，也要注意，蜂蜜虽好，糖尿病人和肝硬化患者不能食用。同时，蜂蜜容易受到肉毒杆菌的污染，可千万不能给一岁之内的宝宝吃。

＼Related information

Honey (Fengmi) has been used as a tonic to nourish and strengthen the body since ancient times. Nowadays, it has become more popular with the improvement of people's living standard. It is included in List of Items That Are both Food and Medicine. As a kind of natural food,

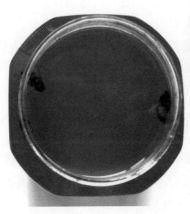

瓶装的蜂蜜，里面还有两只蜜蜂

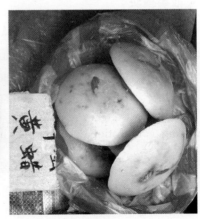

蜂蜡

it has the functions of moistening lung and relieving cough, moistening intestine and relieving constipation, helping sleep, supplementing physical strength and dispelling the effects of alcohol quickly. It can provide nutrition for the body, regulate the effectiveness of various organs, and reduce the occurrence of some common diseases. In addition, honey is often used in beauty products. You can make homemade facial masks using honey and some other materials such as egg white, milk, olive oil and so on. Besides honey, propolis, beeswax, bees, pupae, royal jelly, etc. can also be used as medicine or as health care products.

It should be noted that honey cannot be directly brewed with boiling water; otherwise, the rich vitamins and minerals it contains would be destroyed. It should also be noted that although honey is good, patients with diabetics and cirrhosis cannot take it. At the same time, honey is vulnerable to botulinum toxin contamination, so it must not be given to babies under one year old.

故事模块

在我国，养蜂及蜂产品应用于人类医疗保健的历史悠久。

早在石器时代，人民就已经知道采集树洞、石洞中的蜂蜜等作为食物。中国劳动人民驯养蜜蜂也已有 3000 多年的历史。

同时，古代人们利用蜂蜜、蜂蛹和成虫等蜂产品防治疾病的历史也很悠久。蜂蜜等蜂产品的医用价值在古代的文献和医药专著中有很多记载。下面列举一些仅供参考：

《诗经·周颂·小毖》为我国最早文字记载蜜蜂的资料，告诫人们不要激怒蜜蜂，以免被蜇。东周时期，人们掌握了"以毒攻毒"的理论，开始用蜂蜇治病保健，并将蜂产品用于食品。

我国现存最早的药学专著《神农本草经》将蜂蜜、蜂子和蜂蜡列为上品，并指出了蜂蜜的功效和价值。

汉代医圣张仲景所著的《伤寒杂病论》有蜜蜂制药之例。在《伤寒论》中，记载了用蜂蜜制成栓剂的方法，用来治疗虚弱病人的便秘；还在《金匮要略》中记载了用蜂产品治疗"蛔腹痛"和痢疾的处方。

南北朝时期的陶弘景将蜂蜜进行分类，并指出用蜂蜜等蜂产品美容和保健的作用，能使人"年逾80而壮年"。

著名医药学家孙思邈据说活了102岁。他指出蜂蜜能治咳嗽、气喘、抗衰老，还可用温热蜂蜡外敷治疗扭伤和受风寒引起的腿脚转筋。

明代著名药学家李时珍著《本草纲目》，阐述蜂蜜作为药剂，有五种功效：清热、滋补、解毒、滋润、止痛，并详细记载了蜂产品的治病处方。

由此可见，用蜂蜜及蜂产品进行医疗和保健，既是古代劳动人民智慧的结晶，也是历代医药学家不断探索发现和积累经验的结果。

Story

China has a long history of beekeeping and applying bee products in health care.

As early as the Stone Age, people had known how to collect honey from tree holes and grottos as food. China's working people have been domesticating bees for more than 3,000 years.

Since a long time ago, the ancient people have already begun to use bee products such as honey, pupae and adult bees to prevent and cure diseases. The medical value of bee products such as honey is well documented in ancient literature and medical classics. The following list includes some of the records for readers' reference:

The *Book of Songs* has the earliest written record of bees in China. It warns people not to provoke bees to avoid being stung. During the Eastern Zhou Dynasty, people mastered the theory of "counteracting one toxin with another", and began to treat diseases with bee stings.

They also used bee products for food.

The *Shennong's Classic of Materia Medica*, the earliest existing medical classic in China lists honey, bees and beeswax as top-grade medicines, and points out the efficacy and value of honey.

Zhang Zhongjing, Medical Sage of the Han Dynasty, recorded some examples of bees as a medicine in his *Treatise on Febrile Diseases and Miscellaneous Diseases*. For example, in *Treatise on Febrile Diseases*, the method of making suppository with honey to treat constipation of weak patients is recorded. And the prescriptions of using bee products to treat "abdominal pain due to ascaris" and dysentery are also recorded in *Synopsis of the Golden Chamber*.

During the Northern and Southern Dynasties, Tao Hongjing classified honey and recorded the use of honey and other bee products for beauty and health care. It can make people "healthy even in their eighties".

Sun Simiao, a famous medical scientist, was said to die at the age of 102 years old. He pointed out that honey could cure cough and asthma, and had the anti-aging effect; besides, warm beeswax could be applied to treat sprain and cold-induced cramps in the leg and foot.

Li Shizhen, a famous pharmacologist in the Ming Dynasty, wrote *Compendium of Materia Medica*, explaining that honey as a medicine has five functions: clearing heat, nourishing, detoxifying, moistening and pain relieving. The prescriptions for treating diseases with bee products are also recorded in detail.

It can be seen that the use of honey and bee products for medical treatment and health care is not only the wisdom of the ancient working people, but also the result of continuous exploration, discovery and accumulation of experience by medical scientists of all dynasties in China.

蕲蛇
Qishe / Long-nosed Pit Viper / Agkistrodon

知识模块

来源： 蝰科（Viperidae）动物尖吻腹 *Agkistrodon acutus* (Guenther) 的干燥体。蝰科动物。

产地： 主产于浙江的温州、丽水，江西、福建、湖南、广东亦产。

本草始载： 始载于南北朝《雷公炮炙论》。

功效： 祛风，通络，止痉。

主治： 治疗风湿顽痹、麻木拘挛、中风、半身不遂、破伤风、麻风疥癣。

Basic knowledge

Origin: The dried body of *Agkistrodon acutus* (Guenther) belonging to the family Viperidae.

Location: Qishe is mainly produced in Wenzhou, Lishui of Zhejiang Province; it is also produced in Jiangxi, Fujian, Hunan and Guangdong provinces.

First recorded in: *Lei Gong Pao Zhi Lun* (*Master Lei's Discourse on Drug Processing*) of the Northern and Southern Dynasties.

Efficacy: Dispelling wind, dredging collateral and stopping spasms.

Indications: Rheumatism, numbness, paralysis, stroke, hemiplegia, tetanus and leprosy.

蕲蛇又叫五步蛇，是一种大型的剧毒蛇，属于蝮蛇类。这类蛇所分泌的蛇毒属于血循毒，主要作用于心血管和血液系统。蕲蛇一身都是宝，蛇体可以药用、泡酒，蛇胆、蛇油、蛇蜕、蛇毒等都可以做药材使用。同时蕲蛇也被收载于《既是食品又是药品的物品名单》。

Related information

Qishe is also called Wubushe (five pacer viper). It is a large venomous pit viper species. The venom secreted by these snakes is potent hemotoxin, which mainly acts on cardiovascular and blood systems. Qishe is a treasure. Its body can be soaked for medicinal wine, and its snake gall, snake oil, snake slough, snake venom, etc. can be used as medicine. It is also included in List of Items That Are both Food and Medicine.

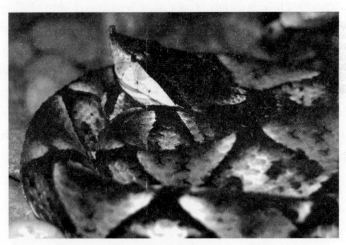

知道"蕲蛇"为什么叫"尖吻腹"吗？看看那个"翘鼻头"

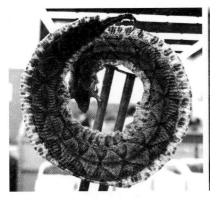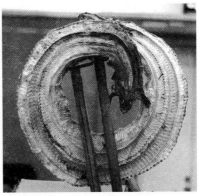

故事模块

　　相传明代嘉靖年间，长沙有个年逾半百的刘员外，家境殷实，膝下只有一女，名叫玉姣，刘员外视其为掌上明珠。

　　玉姣自幼聪慧，因能吟诗作对，而且样貌出众，向她提亲的人络绎不绝，可是她对这些富家公子哥一个都瞧不上，却偏偏爱上了家里年轻英俊又忠厚善良的长工庞生。刘员外气得七窍生烟，将庞生毒打一顿，并把他逐出家门。玉姣偷偷找到庞生，同他拜了天地结为夫妻，一起逃走了。

　　夫妻俩一路奔波，来到了蕲州后，庞生病倒了，只得找了个客栈住下。玉姣卖掉些首饰，请来郎中给庞生诊病。郎中一见庞生患的是麻风病，拒绝为他诊治。店主得知后，就要把他们赶走。玉姣扑通一声跪倒在地，向店主再三苦苦哀求。店主只好让他们搬到客栈后面的一间旧房里住下。

　　很快银两花光了，眼看着庞生的病一天比一天加重，玉姣只好沿街乞讨。一天，玉姣还没有回来，庞生躺在草席上，全身剧痛奇痒，而且饥渴交困，便挣扎着爬起来，正好看见角落里有一个破酒瓮，打开一看，里面有半瓮酒。他喝了一些酒，结果浑身说不出的舒服。于是庞生每天都会喝一些酒瓮里的酒，过了一段时间，庞生的病竟神奇般地好了。

店主得知了这个消息，压根不敢相信，就叫人搬出酒瓮，众人一看，都大吃一惊，只见一条大蕲蛇横卧在瓮中，蛇身已快浸化了。恰巧李时珍从京中归来。他听闻此事，连夜赶来察访，又亲尝了那剩下来的蛇酒，证实了它治病的功效。李时珍十分同情庞生夫妇的遭遇，在玉姣的请求下收了庞生为徒，庞生十分勤奋，不到十年，便名声远扬。

后来，李时珍在撰写《本草纲目》时，特地把蕲蛇酒也写进了。

Story

Legend has it that in Jiajing period of the Ming Dynasty, there was a rich man surnamed Liu who was over fifty years old in Changsha. He had an only daughter named Yujiao. Mr. Liu regarded her as the apple in his eyes.

Yujiao was both talented and good-looking, so many young man wanted to marry her. However, none of them caught the fancy of her. Yujiao fell in love with Pang Sheng, a handsome and kind-hearted young worker in her family. Mr. Liu was so angry that he asked people to beat Pang Sheng up and then drove him out. Yujiao found Pang Sheng and married him secretly. Then they ran away together.

The couple came to Qizhou after a long journey. Pang Sheng fell ill seriously, so they had to settle down in a hotel. Yujiao sold some jewelry and sent for a doctor. The doctor found Pang Sheng was suffering from leprosy, and refused to treat him. Afraid of the horrible disease, the hotel owner tried to drive them out. Yujiao knelt down and implored the hotel owner to keep them. Finally the owner had to let them live in an old and poor hut at the back of the hotel.

Pang Sheng was getting worse and worse, and they had run out of money, so Yujiao had to beg for food in the street. One day, while Yujiao was begging outsides, Pang Sheng, lying on the mat, felt sore and itching all over his body, and he was extremely hungry and thirsty. So he struggled to get up and saw a broken jar in the corner with some alcohol left in it. He drank some wine, and soon he felt much more comfortable. From then on, he would drink some of the wine every day. Gradually his illness was magically cured.

The hotel owner didn't believe it at all when hearing the news. He asked people to take the jar out of the room. Everyone was surprised to see that a large dead Qishe body was curling in the jar, and the snake body was already macerated. At that time Li Shizhen had just returned from Beijing to Qizhou. Hearing about this, Li Shizhen came to visit the couple. He tasted the remaining snake wine and confirmed its effectiveness on the disease. Li Shizhen was very sympathetic to the couple. At the request of Yujiao, he accepted Pang Sheng as his student. Pang Sheng was very diligent and became famous in less than ten years.

Later, when Li Shizhen wrote the *Compendium of Materia Medica*, he specially recorded Qishe wine in it.

麝香
Shexiang / Musk / Moschus

知识模块

来源： 鹿科（Cervidae）动物林麝 *Moschus berezovskii* Flerov、马麝 *M. sifanicus* Przewalski 或原麝 *M. moschiferus* Linnaeus 成熟雄体香囊中的干燥分泌物。

产地： 主产于四川、西藏及云南等地。陕西、甘肃、青海、内蒙古及东北亦产。

本草始载： 始载于东汉《神农本草经》。

功效： 开窍醒神，活血止痛，消肿。

主治： 热病神昏，中风，瘀血证，疮痈肿毒等证。

Basic knowledge

Origin: The dry glandular secretion of mature male *Moschus berezovskii* Flerov, *M. sifanicus* Przewalski or *M. moschiferus* Linnaeus belonging to the family Cervidae.

Location: Shexiang is mainly produced in Sichuan Province, Tibet Autonomous Region and Yunnan Province. It is also produced in Shaanxi, Gansu and Qinghai provinces, Inner Mongolia Autonomous Region and Northeast of China.

First recorded in: *Shenong's Classic of Materia Medica* of the Eastern Han Dynasty.

Efficacy: Inducing resuscitation and refreshing mind, activating blood and alleviating pain, relieving swelling.

Indications: Heat disease and unconsciousness, stroke, blood stasis syndrome, sores, ulcers and abscess.

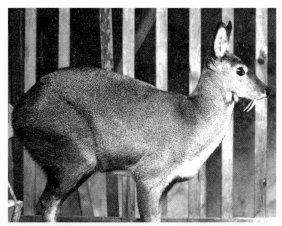

看看这只麝的"獠牙"，这是雄性标志。

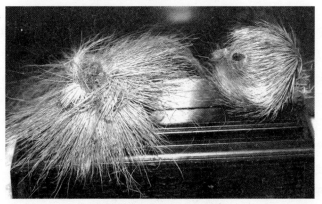

雄麝的香囊，麝香就在里面哦！

拓展模块

麝香本身是雄麝麝香腺分泌物，用来吸引雌麝交配或标记领地，所以只有雄麝才能分泌麝香。判断麝的性别的最简单的办法就是看犬齿，成年的雄麝可见一对上犬齿（俗称獠牙）露出口外。此外，麝香也是著名的天然香料定香剂，被广泛用于高档香水中。

Shexiang is the glandular secretion of male musk deer to attract females to mate or to label the territory, so only the male musk deer can secrete Shexiang. The easiest way to judge the gender of a musk deer is to see whether it has the canine teeth. Adult males have a pair of upper canines (commonly known as tusks). In addition, Shexiang is also a famous perfume fixative, which is widely used in high-grade perfumes.

故事模块

麝香是一味非常名贵的中药，在我国已经有两千多年的药用历史，因其独有的香味和药用价值，被人们称为"中药第一香"。人们在很早就发现了麝香的药用价值，关于麝香的发现，还有一个神奇的传说。

从前，一对唐姓父子居住在深山里，以打猎为生。一天，父子俩在深山老林打猎，儿子为追捕一只野雉，不慎掉下山涧。

儿子虽倒在地上动弹不得，却闻到了不知哪里飘来的缕缕奇香。这奇特的香气，沁人心脾，闻了之后，他的伤痛也好像在逐渐地消散。唐老汉匆匆下来找到儿子，看到儿子闻了香味而伤痛减缓，不由得十分好奇，便四处寻找香气的源头。终于在扒开泥土后发现了一个鸡蛋大小、长着细毛的香囊，香气就是从这个样子奇怪的香囊中散发出来的。在这个香囊的帮助下，不久唐老汉儿子的伤就痊愈了。

唐老汉上山打猎时便加倍留意。他终于发现，雄性麝的腹部有一个囊袋，香味就来源于这个部位，里面分泌出的东西就是"麝香"。

Story

Shexiang is a very valuable Chinese medicine. It has been used for more than two thousand years in China. Because of its unique fragrance and medicinal value, it is called "the first fragrance of Chinese medicines". Its medicinal value has been discovered very early. There is a legend about the discovery of Shexiang.

Once upon a time, an old man surnamed Tang and his son lived in deep mountains, hunting for a living. One day, when they were hunting in the mountains, the son fell carelessly down the mountain stream.

Although the son was unable to move, he smelt some strange fragrance coming from nowhere. The strange fragrance was refreshing, and his pain seemed to be relieved. The old man hurriedly came down to look for his son. When he found that his son was feeling much better due to the fragrance, he was very curious and started to look for the origin of the fragrance. Finally, he dug out an egg-sized fluffy sachet from the soil. The strange fragrance just came from this sachet. Soon the son's injury was cured thanks to this sachet.

The old man paid more attention when he went hunting in the mountains. He finally found that the male musk had a sachet like organ on his abdomen, and the fragrance was just coming from the substance in this sachet. The substance was Shexiang.

四、矿物类 / Mineral medicine

　　矿物药占中药的比例很少，不到整个中药的 1%。矿物药最早起源于道士的炼丹术，但由于很多矿物药含有重金属成分，所以目前常用矿物药不多。现在常用的矿物药有朱砂、石膏、雄黄、芒硝、硫磺、炉甘石、龙骨（动物化石）等。

Mineral medicines account for a small proportion (less than 1%) of Chinese herbal medicine. Mineral medicine originated from Taoist alchemy, but because many mineral medicines contain heavy metals, there are not many mineral medicines nowadays. The commonly used mineral medicines today include cinnabar, gypsum, realgar, mirabilite, sulfur, calamine, Longgu (animal fossils), and so on.

朱砂
Zhusha / Cinnabar / Cinnabaris

知识模块

来源：硫化物类矿物辰砂族辰砂的矿石。

产地：主产于湖南、贵州、四川、云南、广西等地。

本草始载：始载于东汉《神农本草经》。

功效：镇心安神，清热解毒。

主治：治疗心悸易惊，失眠多梦，癫痫，惊风，创疡肿毒等。

Basic knowledge

Origin: The ores of cinnabar belonging to the category of sulphide mineral.

Location: Zhuasha is mainly produced in Hunan, Guizhou, Sichuan, Yunnan provinces, and Guangxi Zhuang Autonomous Region.

First recorded in: *Shenong's Classic of Materia Medica* of the Eastern Han Dynasty

Efficacy: Inducing sedation and tranquilization, clearing heat and relieving toxicity.

Indications: Palpitation, insomnia, epilepsy, infantile convulsions, sores and ulcers, etc.

拓展模块

朱砂在古时多产于辰州（现湖南沅陵），因此也叫辰砂。因其色红，也称为丹砂、赤丹。朱砂性寒，能安神定惊，也有较强的清热解毒作用。现代研究表明，朱砂内服过量可引起中毒，它也被收载于《保健食品禁用物品名单》，因此患者要严格遵医嘱，千万不能擅自服用，甚至久服。而且朱砂不宜入煎剂，此外孕妇、肝肾功能不全者禁用。

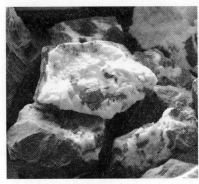

朱砂原矿

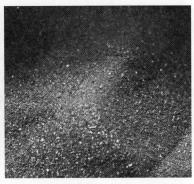

水飞法炮制后的朱砂，非常非常的细

除了药用以外，朱砂在中国传统文化中也占有一席之地。比如传统道教中使用朱砂画符、炼丹、辟邪；风水上来讲，朱砂可以辟邪、镇煞、开运、纳财；中国的传统绘画也被称为"丹青"，丹指丹砂（即朱砂），青指青腂，是两种可作颜料的矿物；再比如，清朝皇帝用朱砂研磨成墨，采用红笔批阅奏折，称为"朱批"。

Related information

In ancient times, Zhusha / cinnabar was mostly produced in Chenzhou (now Yuanling, Hunan Province), so it is also called Chensha. Because of its red color, it is also known as Dansha or Chidan (both "Dan" and "Chi" mean red in Chinese). Cold in nature, Zhusha can calm the nerves and induce tranquilization, and also has a strong effect of clearing heat and toxicity. Modern studies have shown that overdosage of Zhusha can cause poisoning. It is also included in List of Items That Are Prohibited in Health Food. Therefore, patients should strictly follow the doctor's advice and never take it without authorization or even for a long time. Besides, Zhusha should not be used in decoction, and it is forbidden for pregnant women as well as people with liver and kidney dysfunction.

In addition to medicinal use, Zhusha also occupies a place in Chinese traditional culture. For example, in traditional Taoism, Zhusha is used to draw magic figures on paper, or used in alchemy and exorcism; in Chinese feng shui, Zhusha can exorcise and suppress evil spirits, and bring luck or wealth to people; Chinese traditional painting is also known as "Danqing" because of two kinds of minerals often used as pigments-"Dansha" (i.e. Zhusha) and "Qinghuo"; emperors in Qing Dynasty used ink made with ground Zhusha powder to give reply or comment in the reports known as "Zou Zhe" in Chinese handed in by his officials and the emperors' writings are called "Zhupi" (which means reply in red).

故事模块

从前人们普遍都非常迷信，许多人有了病却不去看病求医，而是去找方士。有一种癫狂病，当时的医生们都束手无策，可是有些方士却能治好这种病。因此人们更是"信巫不信医"了。

有个秀才略懂几分医术，他听闻方士能治好癫狂病，心中不禁生疑："方士只会画符念咒，又怎么会真的治病？到底是怎么回事？"他很想弄清楚方士治病的秘密，于是就想出了一个好办法。

这天，秀才让他的媳妇去找方士，说她丈夫得了癫狂病。方士急忙跟着秀才媳妇来到秀才家，只见秀才披头散发、满脸泥污，躺在地上正说疯话呢。

方士一看，秀才果然疯了。他就做好准备要驱"鬼"。方士先端来一碗清水放在桌子上，又拿起一张画好的符，嘴里面还念念有词，然后就要点火烧符，让秀才喝下符水。秀才早有准备，一把抢过符纸，把方士赶了出去。

秀才端起碗喝了口水，发现就是普通的清水，又仔细端详了符纸，也没有发现任何异样，于是反复琢磨，最后，他注意到画符用的朱砂，他想符水能治病，难道是朱砂起到了作用？

第二天，他把一个得癫狂病的人找到自己家，用一点朱砂放在水里给他喝。那人喝了以后，病果然有起色。从此，秀才知道了方士"驱鬼"治癫狂病，只不过因为符上的朱砂有药性。这样，朱砂便成了一味中药。

Story

In the ancient times, people were generally superstitious. Many people did not seek medical treatment when they were ill. They would prefer to go to the alchemists. At that time, a kind of epileptic disease couldn't be cured by doctors but alchemists could cure it. So more and more people chose to believe in alchemists instead of doctors.

There was a scholar who knew something about medicine. When he heard that alchemists could cure the epileptic disease, he was very puzzled. He thought to himself, "Alchemists can do nothing but drawing and chanting incantation. How on earth can they cure people?" Eager to find out the secret of alchemists, he came up with a good idea.

One day, the scholar asked his wife to find an alchemist and told him that her husband was mad due to epileptic. The alchemist rushed to the scholar's house and saw him lying on the ground talking crazily with his hair disheveled and face covered in mud.

The alchemist thought the scholar was really mad, and immediately started his "exorcism ritual". With his mouth murmuring something, the wizard put a bowl of clean water on the table, took out a painted paper, and intended to burn the paper and mix the ashes in the water for the scholar to drink. The scholar suddenly grabbed the paper and drove out the alchemist.

He tasted some water and found that it was just the ordinary clean water. Then he examined the paper but didn't find anything suspicious. So he pondered over and over again. Finally, he noticed the Zhusha that the alchemist used to draw pictures on the paper. He wondered whether it was the Zhusha that cured the disease.

So the next day, he found a mad man and put a little Zhusha in the water for him to drink. After drinking the water, the mad man did show some sign of recovery. The scholar now got the answer to his puzzlement. It was Zhusha that helped alchemist to cure people's epileptic disease during the "exorcism ritual". Therefore, Zhusha became a kind of Chinese herbal medicine.

第三章　中药文化

Culture of Chinese Herbal Medicine

一、古代药学家 / Experts of Chinese Herbal Medicine in Ancient China

　　我国的传统医学源远流长，中医药文化博大精深，在中医药的发展过程中更是名家辈出，他们总结前人经验，不断创新，在救死扶伤的同时也为后人留下了许多经典医药著作，不仅造福一方百姓，而且能福泽子孙后代，对中医药的发展产生了深远的影响。

　　提起古代的中医名家，既有老百姓们最为耳熟能详并带有传奇色彩的神医扁鹊和华佗，也有张仲景、孙思邈、皇甫谧、葛洪、叶天士等中医大家。而中医的发展也离不开历代药学家对中药的研究和积累，中药方面具有突出贡献的名家，当传说中的神农，以及药学家李时珍和孙思邈。

TCM has a long history in China with an extensive and profound culture. In the course of the development of TCM, there are many famous experts. They summarized the experience of their predecessors and innovated constantly. While saving lives, they also left many classic medical works which benefited not only the people at that time, but also the later generations, and had a profound impact on the development of TCM.

When it comes to the famous medical experts in ancient China, the most famous ones are undoubtedly legendary Bian Que and Hua Tuo, who are the most well-known among the common people. Besides, Zhang Zhongjing, Sun Simiao, Huangfu Mi, Ge Hong, Ye Tianshi are also very famous. The development of TCM is also inseparable from the research and accumulation of pharmacists in past dynasties. The legendary Shennong, as well as Li Shizhen and Sun Simiao are certainly the most famous experts of Chinese herbal medicine.

神农/ Shennong

神农尝百草的故事，是一则著名的中国古代神话传说。相传上古时期，人们以打猎和采集野果为生，但有时根本吃不饱，有时则会误食了有毒的东西，当人们生病或中毒的时候，经常无能为力，只能眼巴巴地等待死神的降临。

相传神农为当时的一名部落首领，他看到鸟儿衔种，就发明了五谷农业，并教给大家如何播种五谷，制作农具，大兴水利，使人类能世世代代地生存下去。当他看到部族的人们饱受疾病折磨，于是就亲自尝遍所有的植物，发现哪些植物是有毒的，哪些植物是可以治病的，并用文字记录下这些植物的药性。他为了给百姓治病，不惜冒着生命危险亲身验证植物的药性。古书中记载"神农尝百草，一日遇七十毒"，就是神农氏的不畏艰难险阻，勇于探索，以及伟大的自我牺牲精神的真实写照。

《神农本草经》是中医四大经典著作之一，也是现存最早的中药学专著。它的作者不详，一般认为成书于东汉时期，是秦汉时期众多医学家搜集、整理、总结当时药物学经验成果的专著，是对中国中医药的第一次系统总结。既然作者不是神农，为什么还要以神农的名义给书命名呢？原来，它是希望借用当时妇孺皆知的神农尝百草的传说以及神农的名字，来提高它的知名度和地位。

《神农本草经》全书分三卷，记载了 365 种药物（其中植物药252 种，动物药 67 种，矿物药46 种），分为上、中、下三品，对每一味药的产地、性质、采集时间、入药部位和主治病症都有详细记载。在李时珍出版《本草纲目》之前，该书一直被看作是最权威的医书。

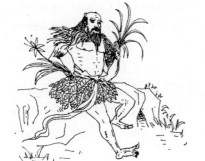

神农

"Shennong tasted hundreds of medicinal herbs" is a famous myth from ancient China. Legend has it that in ancient times, people hunted animals and gathered wild fruits for a living, but sometimes they did not have enough to eat, and sometimes they would even eat poisonous things by mistake. When people were sick or got poisoned, they could do nothing but wait for death.

According to the legend, Shennong was a tribal leader at that time. When he saw the birds holding seeds in their beaks, he invented agriculture. Then he started to teach his people how to sow the grains, make farm tools, and develop water conservancy, so that mankind could survive from generation to generation. When he saw people in his tribe suffering from diseases, he tasted all the herbs by himself in order to find out which herbs were poisonous and which herbs were able to cure people. He also recorded the medicinal properties of these herbs. In order to cure his people, he even risked his own life to verify the medical effects of these herbs in person. "When Shennong tasted herbs, he got poisoned seventy times in a single day", as described in ancient books, is a true portrayal of his courage and self-sacrifice.

Shennong's Classic of Materia Medica is one of the four classics of TCM. It is also one of the earliest monographs of Chinese medicines. Its author is unknown. It is generally believed that the book was written in the Eastern Han Dynasty (25−220). Many medical experts in the Qin and Han Dynasties collected, sorted out and summarized a lot of medical achievements and experience, resulting in this classic work. It can be seen as the first systematic summary of TCM. Since the author is not Shennong, why was the book in the name of him? Actually, it relied on the legend of Shennong who was known to the common people at that time in order to improve its popularity among the general public.

Divided into three volumes, the book lists 365 medicines (including 252 botanical medicines, 67 animal medicines and 46 mineral medicines). The medicines are graded into upper, middle and low herbs. The origin, nature, collection time, medicinal parts and the main diseases they can treat are all recorded in detail. Before Li Shizhen published the *Compendium of Materia Medica*, *Shennong's Classic of Materia Medica* has always been regarded as the most authoritative medical book in ancient China.

李时珍 / Li Shizhen

李时珍（1518—1593）是明代著名医药学家。他家世代行医，但当时民间医生地位很低，于是父亲决定让李时珍读书应考，希望他能够出人头地。但李时珍屡次落第，便决心放弃科举专心学医。没几年，李时珍就成为很有名望的医生，还被推荐上京任太医院判，但是由于看不惯官场的乌烟瘴气，只任职一年，他便辞职回乡。李时珍阅读了大量古医籍，又经过临床实践发现古代的本草书籍错误百出，于是他决心要重新编纂一部本草书籍。

在编写《本草纲目》的过程中李时珍遇到了许多困扰，同时也认识到，"读万卷书"固然需要，但"行万里路"更不可少，需要深入实地进行调查才行。他跋山涉水，遍访名医宿儒，搜求民间验方，观察和收集药物标本，足迹遍布湖广、江西、江苏、安徽等许多地方。李时珍非常注意观察药物的形态和生长情况，而且并不满足于走马看花式的调查，而是对着实物进行比较核对。

就这样，李时珍经过长期艰苦的实地调查，搞清了许多疑难问题，于公元1578年完成了《本草纲目》的编写工作。全书约有190万字，52卷，载药1892种，在前人基础上新增药物374种，记录一万多个药方，附

图一千多幅，成了我国药物学的空前巨著。书中纠正了许多前人的错误，在动植物分类学等许多方面有突出成就，并对其他有关的学科（如生物学、化学、矿物学、地质学、天文学等）也做出了巨大贡献。达尔文称赞它是"中国古代的百科全书"。

Li Shizhen (1518-1593) is a famous medical scientist in the Ming Dynasty. His family practiced medicine for generations, but at that time the doctors were not highly respected, so his father decided to let Li Shizhen study for the imperial examination, hoping that he could have a promising future. But after several consecutive failures, Li Shizhen decided to give up the imperial examination and concentrate on learning medicine instead. Within a few years, Li Shizhen became a well-known doctor and was appointed as the head doctor for the royal family. However, being tired of officialdom, he resigned and returned home after only one year. Back at home, Li Shizhen read a lot of ancient medical books, and after a lot of clinical practice, he found that these books were full of mistakes, so he decided to re-compile a medicinal book himself.

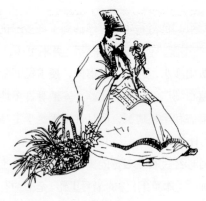

李时珍

In the process of compiling *Compendium of Materia Medica*, Li Shizhen came across many troubles. He realized that "reading ten thousand volumes of books" is necessary, but "traveling ten thousand miles" is even more indispensable since field trip was more important than books. Therefore, he traveled mountains and rivers, visited famous doctors and scholars, searched folk prescriptions, observed and collected drug specimens, and traveled all over many places of China. Li Shizhen paid great attention to the morphology and growth of the herbs. Not satisfied with the desultory survey, he thought it important to compare and check the real herbs.

In this way, after a long and arduous field investigation, Li Shizhen solved many difficult problems and completed the compilation of *Compendium of Materia Medica* in 1578 AD. The book contains about 1.9 million words, 52 volumes and 1,892 medicines. 374 new medicines were added, more than 10,000 prescriptions were recorded and more than 1,000 drawings were attached in the book, which made it an unprecedented masterpiece of pharmacology in China. Besides correcting many mistakes of the predecessors, the book has made outstanding achievements in taxonomy of animals and plants, and also has made great contributions to other related disciplines, such as biology, chemistry, mineralogy, geology, astronomy and so on. Darwin praised it as "an encyclopedia in ancient China".

孙思邈 / Sun Simiao

孙思邈是唐代杰出的医药学家，被后人尊称为"药王"。他是一位富有传奇色彩的人物，生于541年或581年，卒于682年，虽然他的出生年月尚无定论，但他年逾百岁确是高寿。

孙思邈自幼多病，耗尽家财求医看病，因此立志于学习医学。他从小就天资聪颖，被称为"圣童"，长大后不仅医术精湛为乡邻看病，而且精通道家老庄学说和佛家经典著作。孙思邈渐渐获得了很高的声名，但他无心追逐仕途功名，屡次拒绝隋文帝、唐太宗、唐高宗入仕为官的邀请，而选择隐居山林，研究医学和养生之道，并采药行医，济世救民。

孙思邈医术精湛，非常重视民间医疗经验，但不墨守成规，出色地发展了仲景学说。他流传下来的《千金要方》和《千金翼方》两本著作，最为后世称道。

《千金要方》又名《备急千金要方》或《千金方》，成书于652年，全书三十卷，合方论五千三百首。书中首篇所列的《大医精诚》是论述医德的一篇重要文献，被誉为是"东方的希波克拉底誓言"。书中收集

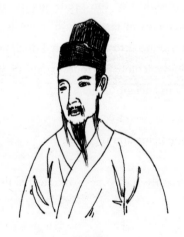

孙思邈

了从张仲景时代直至孙思邈的临床经验，历数百年的方剂成就，是对唐代以前中医学成就的一次很好的总结，对后世医学特别是方剂学的发展，有着重要的影响，堪称中国最早的医学百科全书。

《千金翼方》是孙思邈晚年著作，是对《千金要方》的全面补充。全书三十卷，合方、论、法二千九百余首，内容涉及本草、妇人、伤寒、小儿、养性、补益、中风、杂病、疮痈以及针灸等各个方面，尤以治疗伤寒、中风、杂病和疮痈最见疗效。书中收载的800余种药物当中，有200余种详细介绍了有关药物的采集和炮制等相关知识。

Sun Simiao was an outstanding medical scientist in Tang Dynasty who was honored as the "King of Medicine" by later generations. He was a legendary figure born in 541 or 581 and died in 682. Although the date of his birth has not been confirmed yet, what is certain is that he lived to over 100 years old.

Sun Simiao was often sick when he was a little child, and his family spent all their money seeking medical treatment for him, so he was determined to study medicine. He was an intelligent boy, known as the "holy boy". When he grew up, he was not only able to treat his neighbors with excellent medical skills, but also had a good knowledge of Chinese Taoist Theory and Buddhist classics. Sun Simiao gradually gained a high reputation, but he did not intend to pursue official career and fame. He repeatedly refused the invitation of emperors to work in the royal court. Instead, he chose to live in seclusion in the mountains where he studied medicine and regimen, and practiced medicine to save people.

Sun Simiao not only had superb medical skill, but also attached great importance to folk medical experience. He did not stick to the convention; instead, he developed Zhongjing's theory excellently. *Qian Jin Yao Fang (Recipes Worth A Thousand Gold)* and *Qian Jin Yi Fang (A*

Supplement to Recipes Worth A Thousand Gold) are two of his works that survived to this day and were always praised by later generations.

Qian Jin Yao Fang, also known as *Beiji Qian Jin Yao Fang* or *Qian Jin Fang*, was finished in 652. It is composed of 30 volumes, including 5300 discourses on preion. The text On the Absolute Sincerity of Great Physicians is an important document on medical ethics, often called "the Chinese Hippocratic Oath". The book collects the clinical experience from the era of Zhang Zhongjing to his time, and the good prescriptions in the past hundreds of years. It is a good summary of the achievements of TCM before the Tang Dynasty. It has great influence upon the development of Chinese Medicine in later generations, especially prescriptions of TCM. It can be called the earliest medical encyclopedia in China.

Qian Jin Yi Fang, another book written in his later life, is a comprehensive supplement to *Qian Jin Yao Fang*. This book is composed of 30 volumes, including more than 2900 discourses on preion, covering various aspects such as herbal medicines, women's diseases, typhoid fever, children's diseases, self-cultivation, tonic, stroke, miscellaneous diseases, sores, acupuncture and moxibustion and so on, especially in the treatment of typhoid fever, stroke, miscellaneous diseases and sores. More than 800 herbal medicines are included in the book, and more than 200 medicines of them are introduced in detail including the relevant knowledge of collection and processing of medicines.

二、中国四大药都 / Four "Medicine Capitals" of China

　　我国的中医药历史悠久，伴随着中医文化的不断发展，中药文化也历经数千年发展至今，已经发展出了成熟的体系，出现了四大规模化、专业化的药材城市，安徽亳州、河北安国、江西樟树和河南禹州，并称为中国四大药都。

China's TCM has a long history. With the development of TCM, the culture of Chinese herbal medicine has developed into a mature system after thousands of years. Four large-scale and specialized cities of medicinal materials, Bozhou of Anhui Province, Anguo of Hebei Province, Zhangshu of Jiangxi Province and Yuzhou of Henan Province, have emerged. They are known as China's four major "medicine capitals".

亳州 / Bozhou

　　四大药都之首亳州位于安徽省，相传汉代名医华佗就出生于这里，正因如此，亳州的医药业发展迅速，早在明清时期，亳州就已经药商云集，药铺林立，药市非常繁荣，是闻名天下的药都之一。发展到今天，它已经成为全国最大的药材集散地和价格形成中心，拥有全球规模最大的中药材交易中心，年销售收入突破百亿元。亳州也是著名的中药材种植基地，有不少中药是以亳州的"亳"而冠名的，比如亳菊、亳白芍等。

Bozhou, the top of the four medicine capitals, is located in Anhui Province. It is known as the hometown of Hua Tuo and hometown of medicinal materials. Hua Tuo, a famous doctor of Han Dynasty, was

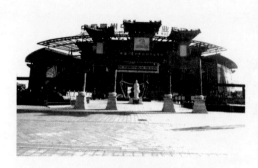

亳州中药材市场

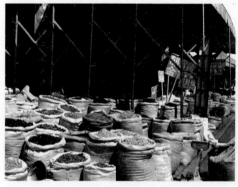

市场内药材种类齐全

born here. Because of this, the pharmaceutical industry of Bozhou developed rapidly. As early as the Ming and Qing Dynasties, Bozhou was already rather famous for the prosperous medicine market that was full of herbal medicine shops. Today, it has become the largest distribution center and price formation center of Chinese medicinal materials in China, with the largest trading center of Chinese medicinal materials in the world with annual sales exceeding 10 billion yuan. Bozhou is also a famous planting base of Chinese herbal medicines. Many Chinese medicines are named with Bo, such as Bo-Juhua, Bo-Baishao and so on.

安国 / Anguo

　　河北省的安国是我国北方最大的中药材集散地和中药文化发祥地，素以"药都"和"天下第一药市"享誉海内外。安国古称祁州，盛产药材历史悠久，出产祁菊花、祁山药等八大祁药。这里的中药材交易已有千年历史，始于北宋，盛于明清，享有"草到安国方成药，药经祁州始生香"的美誉。目前安国药市已被列入首批国家非物质文化遗产名录，这里的药王庙和安国中药文化博物馆也是全国重点文物保护单位。元代著名戏剧家关汉卿就是诞生于此。

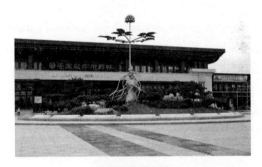

安国中药材市场

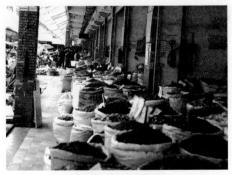

药材市场内商家云集

265

Anguo of Hebei Province is the largest distribution center of Chinese medicinal materials and the birthplace of Chinese medicine culture in northern China. It is known both at home and abroad as "medicine capital" and "the world's first medicine market". Anguo was called Qizhou in ancient times, and it has a long history of medicinal herbs planting, such as the famous "eight Chinese herbal medicines with the name of Qi", including Qi-Juhua and Qi-Shanyao. The trade of Chinese medicines here has a history of thousands of years. It began in the Northern Song Dynasty and flourished in the Ming and Qing Dynasties. Therefore, there is a saying popular here "Herbs can become medicines only when they come to Qizhou; medicines can get fragrance only when they come to Qizhou". At present, the medicine market in Anguo has been listed in the first batch of National Intangible Cultural Heritage List. Besides, Temple of the God of Medicine and the Anguo Museum of Traditional Chinese Medicine Culture are also national key cultural relic protection units. Guan Hanqing, a famous dramatist of the Yuan Dynasty, was born here.

樟树 / Zhangshu

　　江西省的樟树在历史上曾叫清江县，与瓷都景德镇等并称江西四大古镇，又因"聂友射鹿"的传奇故事而得名樟树。樟树的药业源远流长，是我国历史上最大的药材集散地之一，距今已有1800多年的历史。现在它以其特有的药材生产、加工、炮制和经营闻名遐迩，素享"药不到樟树不齐，药不过樟树不灵"之美誉，是我国著名的南国药都。

Historically, the Zhangshu of Jiangxi Province was called Qingjiang County. It was one of the four ancient towns in Jiangxi together with other three towns including Jingdezhen, the porcelain capital. It was named Zhangshu because of the legendary story of "Nieyou shooting deer". It has been over 1800 years since Zhangshu became one of the largest distribution centers of medicinal materials. Now it is well-known for cultivation, processing and operation of medicinal materials. There is a saying popular here "Medicines are not enough before they come to Zhangshu; medicines are not effective before they come to Zhangshu". It is the famous medicine capital of South China.

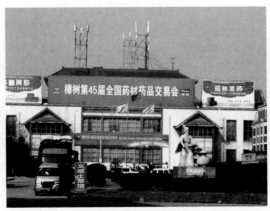

樟树中药材市场

禹州 / Yuzhou

河南省的禹州是古代大禹治水的地方，曾是我国第一个王朝夏朝的都城，时称阳翟。禹州素有"中华药城"之称，也是我国医药发祥地之一。禹州有悠久的中药材种植、采集、加工历史，以加工精良、遵古炮制著称于世，据传自春秋战国以来，扁鹊、张仲景、孙思邈等都曾在这里行医采药、著书立说。在他们的影响下，禹州的医药业也得到大的发展，从唐朝开始，药市逐步形成，明朝时期，禹州就成为全国药材集散地之一。

Yuzhou of Henan Province was the place where Dayu combated the flood in ancient times. It was the capital of the Xia Dynasty, the first dynasty in China. It was called Yangdi at that time. Yuzhou is known as the "Chinese Medicine City" and one of the birthplaces of Chinese medicine. Yuzhou has a long history of planting, collecting and processing Chinese medicinal materials. It is known for its excellent processing of medicines, especially ancient processing methods. It is said

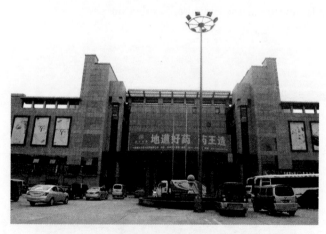

禹州中药材市场

that since the Spring and Autumn Period and the Warring States Period, Bian Que, Zhang Zhongjing, Sun Simiao and some other famous medical experts in history have practiced medicine, collected medicinal herbs and wrote medical books here. Under their influence, Yuzhou's pharmaceutical industry has developed quickly. From the Tang Dynasty, the pharmaceutical market was gradually formed. During the Ming Dynasty, Yuzhou became one of the national distribution centers of Chinese herbal medicine.

三、诺贝尔奖与中药现代化 / Nobel Prize and Modernization of Chinese Herbal Medicine

2015 年 10 月 5 日，诺贝尔奖委员会在瑞典斯德哥尔摩宣布，将 2015 年诺贝尔生理学和医学奖授予中国女科学家屠呦呦和一名日本科学家及一名爱尔兰科学家，以表彰他们在寄生虫疾病治疗研究中取得的成就。这是中国科学家凭借在中国本土进行的科学研究而首次获诺贝尔科学奖，是中国医学界迄今为止获得的最高奖项，也是中医药成果获得的最高奖项。

On October 5, 2015, the Nobel Prize Committee announced in Stockholm, Sweden that it would award the Nobel Prize in Physiology or Medicine 2015 to Tu Youyou, a Chinese female scientist, a Japanese scientist and an Irish scientist for their achievements in the treatment of parasitic diseases. This is the first time that Chinese scientists have won the Nobel Prize for their scientific research in China. It is the highest award ever won by the Chinese medical community and the highest prize for the achievements of TCM.

屠呦呦，1930 年 12 月 30 日于出生于浙江省宁波市，是一位药学家。20 世纪六七十年代，在极为艰苦的科研条件下，屠呦呦率领的中国中医科学院团队从系统收集历代医籍、地方药志和名老中医经验入手，汇集了 2000 多种方药，从中筛选出 200 多种供筛选，最后从东晋葛洪所著的《肘后备急方》中对青蒿治疗疟疾的描述"青蒿一握，以水二升渍，绞取汁"中得到启发，把原来高温煎煮的方法改为了用低沸点溶剂乙醚来提取其中的有效成分，从青蒿中提取出了青蒿素，从而开创了疟疾治

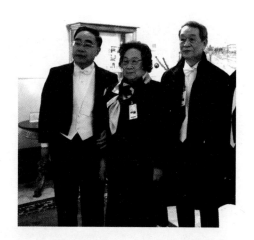

屠呦呦（中）在丈夫（右）和中国中医科学院院长、天津中医药大学校长张伯礼院士（左）陪同下在瑞典领奖。

疗新方法，全球数亿人因这种"中国神药"而受益。凭借青蒿素的发现，屠呦呦也由此成为迄今第一位获得诺贝尔科学奖的本土中国科学家、第一位获得诺贝尔生理医学奖的华人科学家，由此实现了中国人在自然科学领域诺贝尔奖零的突破。

Tu Youyou, born in Ningbo, Zhejiang Province on December 30, 1930, is a pharmacist. In the 1960s and 1970s, under extremely difficult scientific research conditions, Tu Youyou lead a team of China Academy of Chinese Medical Sciences, and they collected more than 2000 prescriptions from medical books, medical chorography and the experience of famous Chinese medicine experts. More than 200 prescriptions were further screened out. Finally, she was inspired by the description of using Qinghao (sweet wormwood herb) to treat malaria in *Zhouhou Beiji Fang* (*The Handbook of Prescriptions for Emergencies*) written by Ge Hong in the Eastern Jin Dynasty: "Soak a handful of sweet wormwood herb in two liters of water, then mash and filter the

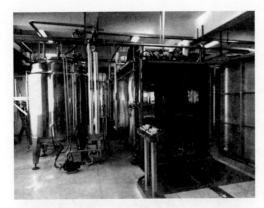

现代化的制药设备

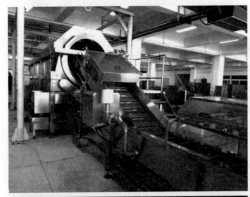

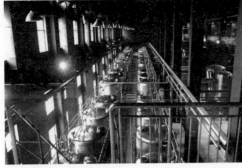

现代化的制药车间

liquid." Therefore, the method of high temperature decoction was replaced by ether, a low boiling point solvent, to extract active ingredients from sweet wormwood herb. In this way, artemisinin was extracted, thus creating a new treatment for malaria. Hundreds of millions of people around the world benefited from this "magic medicine from China". With the discovery of artemisinin, Tu Youyou became the first native Chinese scientist to win the Nobel Prize for Science and the first Chinese scientist to win the Nobel Prize for Physiology and Medicine, thus achieving a breakthrough in the field of natural science in China.

屠呦呦用现代科学方法促进了中医药传承和创新，把中医药推向世界，她获得诺贝尔奖，也是中药现代化的胜利，为我国的中医药的创新发展带来了巨大的信心和鼓舞，为中药现代化带来巨大启示。

我国的中医药学就像一个珍贵的宝库，里面蕴含着像青蒿素一样可以造福全人类的宝藏，正等待着我们去发现、挖掘。但由于缺乏科学系统的阐述和先进的技术方法，对中药作用机理、物质基础等方面的研究还不够深入，一直以来中药难以得到世界的认可，因此急需通过中药现代化来解决这些问题。中药现代化就是指在继承和发扬传统中医药的优势和特色的基础上，依靠现代先进科学技术手段，遵守严格的规范标准，研究出高效、安全、稳定、可控的现代中药产品，达到国际主流市场标准，可以在国际上广泛流通。屠呦呦成功研制出青蒿素说明中药现代化的方向是正确的，这为中药产业未来的发展树立了一个良好的榜样。

令人欣喜的是，2016年12月25日《中华人民共和国中医药法》颁布，这是中医药的第一部国家法律。其施行是为了继承和弘扬中医药文化，保障和促进中医药事业发展，是中医药事业发展史上重要的里程碑！

虽然在未来中医药走向世界面临着许多竞争和挑战，但相信我国的中医药事业必定会有长足的发展，造福世界上更多的人类。

Tu Youyou promoted the inheritance and innovation of TCM with modern scientific methods. She also pushed TCM to the world. Her winning the Nobel Prize means the victory of the modernization of Chinese pharmaceutical industry, which brought confidence and inspiration to the innovation and development of TCM in China, and also brought great inspiration to the modernization of Chinese herbal medicine.

TCM of China is like a precious treasure house full of treasures like artemisinin which can benefit all mankind. They are waiting for us to discover and excavate. However, due to the lack of scientific and systematic elaboration and advanced technology and methods, the research on the mechanism and material basis of Chinese herbal medicine is not deep enough. It has been difficult for Chinese herbal medicine to be recognized by the world. Therefore, it is urgent to solve these problems through the modernization of Chinese herbal medicine. On the basis of inheriting and developing the advantages and characteristics of Chinese herbal medicine, relying on modern advanced scientific and technological means and abiding by strict standards, the modernization of Chinese herbal medicine refers to the research of modern Chinese medicine products with high efficiency, safety, stability and controllability, which can reach the international mainstream market standards and can be widely circulated in the world. Tu Youyou's successful extracting of artemisinin shows that the direction of modernization of Chinese herbal medicine is correct, and also sets a good example for the future development of Chinese pharmaceutical industry.

It is gratifying that on December 25, 2016, *Law of the People's Republic of China on Traditional Chinese Medicine* was promulgated. It is the first national law on TCM. Its implementation is to inherit and carry forward the culture of TCM, and ensure and promote the development of TCM. It is indeed an important milestone in the history of the development of TCM.

Although there are many challenges for TCM in the future, we firmly believe that the cause of TCM in China will surely have great development and benefit more people in the whole world.